# HEALING
# SIBO

# HEALING
# SIBO

### Fix the Real Cause of IBS, Bloating, and Weight Issues in 21 Days

## SHIVAN SARNA

AVERY

*an imprint of Penguin Random House*
*New York*

**AVERY**

an imprint of Penguin Random House LLC
penguinrandomhouse.com

Most Avery books are available at special quantity discounts for bulk purchase for sales promotions, premiums, fund-raising, and educational needs. Special books or book excerpts also can be created to fit specific needs. For details, write SpecialMarkets@penguinrandomhouse.com.

Library of Congress Cataloging-in-Publication Data

Names: Sarna, Shivan, author.
Title: Healing SIBO: Fix the real cause of IBS, bloating, and weight issues in 21 days / Shivan Sarna.
Description: New York: Avery, an imprint of Penguin Random House, [2021] | Includes index.
Identifiers: LCCN 2020034728 (print) | LCCN 2020034729 (ebook) | ISBN 9780593191774 (paperback) | ISBN 9780593191781 (ebook)
Subjects: LCSH: Gastrointestinal system—Diseases—Popular works. | Self-care, Health—Popular works.
Classification: LCC RC801 .S17 2021 (print) | LCC RC801 (ebook) | DDC 616.3/3—dc23
LC record available at https://lccn.loc.gov/2020034728
LC ebook record available at https://lccn.loc.gov/2020034729
p.    cm.

Printed in the United States of America


Book design by Silverglass

To anyone who has ever had a medical mystery

# CONTENTS

# Foreword

I first met Shivan Sarna when her name appeared on my list of tele-medicine appointments one day. Initially, Shivan knew almost nothing about SIBO except that she had it and whatever she'd been able to find out from Dr. Google. But she was totally committed to educating herself. For a while, we were meeting virtually (in both senses of the word) every week, and it soon became clear that we had a similar mission—to learn as much as possible about SIBO, spread that knowledge, and raise awareness about this condition, which was (and still is) actually unknown to the vast majority of people both in and out of the medical profession.

We started working together to fulfill this mission with a series of free online SIBO Summits. When Shivan first told me she was planning to hold an online health summit about SIBO, I was eager to help. At first, I introduced her to experts in the field, convinced them to talk to her, and helped her formulate the questions to ask them. But after the first season, she didn't need me to do any of those things anymore. Now, she's interviewed almost everyone who knows anything about SIBO and has become an expert herself. I started out as her doctor but quickly became her educational partner and friend.

Shivan is uniquely qualified to write a book for the general reader about SIBO and its relation to IBS because of the simple fact that she is *not* a doctor. A book written by a medical professional wouldn't include all the invaluable, personal, nonmedical information and advice that really has to come from the perspective of the educated patient. In this book she not only consolidates all the cutting-edge technical information she's learned from doctors and nutritionists, but she also walks her readers through the emotional, psychological, and very practical issues they have to navigate and negotiate living with SIBO on a daily basis. Shivan also brings a unique perspective as a vegetarian and shares how to navigate SIBO healing with plant-based foods.

It is vitally important to provide this information to as many people as possible, because it has been estimated that up to one billion people around the world have IBS, and up to 78 percent of those IBS cases have been caused by SIBO. And yet, despite these staggering numbers, SIBO has been underfunded and under-researched. Because it affects so many people and so often goes undiagnosed, SIBO desperately needs all the attention it can get. So thank you, Shivan, for sharing what you've learned as well as your favorite recipes and your practical advice. I truly believe that you are performing an invaluable service and giving hope to millions of people with this book.

—*Allison Siebecker, ND, MSOM, LAc*

# My Story and an Overview of the Plan

I was in the bathroom sweating. It was close to three o'clock. I'd just finished lunch with my boss at a really fabulous restaurant, and I had to go to the ladies' room. I hope you don't know what I mean when I say I really "had to go," but if you're reading this book, you probably do.

In fact, I've actually heard worse "tales from the ladies' room." One of my friends can't drive for more than twenty minutes without having to use the bathroom, which severely limits the routes she is able to take. There are also families who haven't seen relatives in years because they're afraid to be on a plane without instant access to the facilities.

In that instance, I was in the bathroom that day for at least twenty minutes. This was before cell phones, and I knew that my boss and our waiter must have been wondering what had happened to me.

When I finally got out of there the waiter looked worried, and my poor boss, a polite man in his forties, asked me if I was all right. What could I say? I just mumbled something about being sorry and said "body functions" and shrugged my shoulders. Truthfully, I was completely mortified and just wished I could disappear. My goal that day had been to ask for a raise, but clearly that wasn't happening. He settled the bill and we left. It was awkward, to say the least, and all these years later, I still remember it.

\* \* \* \*

I call my experience as a person with SIBO the journey of a lifetime because I remember having symptoms starting as far back as the age of four—even though I certainly had no idea what was causing them.

Back then, our family had pizza for dinner every Friday night, and most of those nights I threw up after dinner. My magnificent mother was taking care of three young daughters; she was tired, and she just wanted something that was good and fast for dinner at the end of a busy week. She knew that I wasn't really sick; I wasn't getting stomach flu every Friday evening. And she would have been horrified if anyone thought she was being a bad mother. In fact, I actually loved pizza night. I liked it enough going down that I was willing to tolerate throwing it up—and it didn't happen every single time. Still, it should have been more of a warning sign than either of us realized.

My father, however, was from India and well-versed in the principles of Ayurvedic medicine, the ancient healing science of India, which include building and maintaining a healthy metabolic system (the conversion of food into fuel for your body) through good digestion and excretion. According to Ayurveda, regular, healthy bowel movements are a major indicator of good digestion and, therefore, overall health. So, when he noticed that I wasn't "going" every day, he mentioned it to my mother, who began to question me about the quantity and quality of my poops. Even at that early age, I already felt this was none of my mom's business. Although I now understand that my parents were concerned about my chronic constipation, as a five- or six-year-old, I resented being questioned about my bathroom habits and having to sit on the toilet for what seemed to me inordinate lengths of time day in and day out. That is actually one of my earliest memories.

And those weren't the only gastrointestinal issues that appeared very early in my life. By the time I was eight years old, I'd been to India four times on buying trips with my parents, who were importers of Indian art and handicrafts, and I suspect that on one or more of those trips I must have had some kind of food poisoning, which I now know is most often the primary cause of SIBO. Unfortunately, neither of my parents is still alive, so I really have no one to confirm my suspicion, but it seems logical. Basically, I was just a skinny kid who was always constipated, with a big bloated belly and a sensitive stomach. But I just thought that was normal.

In middle school and high school I was uncomfortable a lot of the time, and my friends sometimes affectionately referred to my tummy as my Buddha belly, but for the most part—aside from one bad bout with mononucleosis—I was too busy being a teenager to pay much attention to my symptoms.

Luckily, because of my father's knowledge of Ayurvedic medicine, which depends heavily on diet and herbal cures, and the fact that my mother was an early advocate of natural healing, I was brought up to follow a clean diet. By the time I was in my twenties I had given up eating meat and drinking alcohol, and I started to meditate. All of this put me on the spiritual path I follow to this day, and I've had more than one doctor tell me that if I hadn't been following such a clean lifestyle, I'd probably have been even sicker.

You'd think that I'd want to get to the root of what was causing all my unpleasant, often painful symptoms and try to get rid of them once and for all, but actually it took decades. For a long time, I might mention my bathroom issues to a doctor in passing, but he or she never seemed to think my symptoms were worth serious consideration, and I certainly didn't discuss my elimination habits with my friends. It's a taboo subject, but we need to talk about it, especially if there is a problem. But those of us who suffer from SIBO don't even realize we are experiencing a true health issue because we have become so used to our symptoms that they feel "normal." We think we just have a "delicate" or a "sensitive" stomach.

At that point in my life, I was a successful yoga teacher. Shivan's Yoga Studio was a hotspot for healing in Sarasota, Florida. I even had my own television program, and I traveled around the world speaking to women about how to hone their managerial skills. I loved the work, and I felt really good about helping so many people. But while there are people who actually thrive on traveling, being on the road so much of the time was wreaking havoc with my health—to the point where I knew I just couldn't do it anymore. This was in the '90s. I was a vegetarian at a time when restaurants didn't know what to do with plant-based eaters, and, therefore, I ate enough pasta primavera to last for the rest of my life. I was anxious about my home and the kitties I was leaving behind every week. It was not a sustainable lifestyle for me. Plus, I was losing my hair from the stress and I was germophobic from being on so many planes and staying in so many hotel rooms.

That's when my best friend and spiritual teacher suggested I become a host on what was then called the Home Shopping Network. I thought they were nuts, but, serendipitously, I met a woman at a seminar shortly thereafter who worked at HSN. It seemed to me that the Universe had put her in my path, so I went for an interview, and that meeting turned out to be the pivotal event that changed my life forever. Six months later I got the job. It fit my skill set perfectly, and it was great that I could sleep in my own bed, be with my cats, and see my friends. For the first six years, I was assigned the overnight shift. I drove an hour to work in the evening, got that adrenaline rush from appearing on TV, and then drove home and tried to sleep during the day. Needless to say, this schedule, plus the pressures of the work itself, really messed up my circadian rhythm, and the lack of sleep was wreaking havoc with my health. The perfect storm was brewing.

I'd been feeling sick and dealing with a bloated belly even though I was working out and eating well. Forcing yourself into slim wear to be on television every day so that America doesn't wonder if you are pregnant is not a stress I would wish on anyone. So, I finally went to see a gastroenterologist, who diagnosed me with irritable bowel syndrome. IBS is a "functional disorder," meaning that the symptoms are real but doctors can't find any obvious cause for them. This makes it really difficult to treat. How do you cure something that isn't being caused by anything?

He then prescribed an antidepressant, which was not only discouraging but also confusing and extremely frustrating. I quite naturally assumed he was telling me that it was all in my head while I knew it wasn't. I now understand that he was trying to raise my serotonin levels, because the majority of the serotonin in your system is actually made and stored in your gut, and it plays a significant role in regulating gastrointestinal function. But I didn't know that then, and this doctor did not explain his reasoning to me. He also suggested that running three miles a day would help, but at that point I didn't have the time or energy for exercise. I was living on Maalox to calm my acid reflux, taking Benadryl to help me get to sleep, and sleeping twelve hours a day just to have enough energy to do the overnight shows for HSN.

I'd already suspected that I might have IBS because I'd seen a Netflix documentary about it, and, having been into health food and yoga since I was a teenager, I thought I knew what to do. I was eating a textbook "healthy" diet—plant-based foods like whole grains and lots of fruits and veggies, so I didn't understand why I still felt so bad. I'd eat an apple thinking it was good for me, not knowing that what was healthy for someone else wouldn't work for me at all.

The harder I tried to "be healthy," the worse I felt—what with the fatigue and the fact that my gastrointestinal problems were getting worse and worse. I realized it wasn't just random symptoms but a pattern, and I began to get scared—very scared—thinking I might have cancer or some other devastating illness.

I'm normally a very social person. I loved meeting friends for lunch, but, because I was so exhausted and felt so sick, on a regular basis I was starting to cancel plans I had made. I was pretty much just working, sleeping, and doing the bare minimum to stay afloat. I was alive but not really living, and I knew I couldn't keep going the way I was. I needed to get to the bottom of this once and for all.

I went back to the doctor and had more testing done, trying to rule out anything more serious than IBS. I had virtually every kind of scope you could think of—colonoscopy, endoscopy—basically, if it ended in "oscopy," I did the procedure. All my tests came back negative. I felt worse than ever, and I wasn't getting any closer to an answer for my problem.

When I finally got tested for SIBO it was almost by accident. I had a work friend at the time who had similar gastrointestinal issues and who was also gluten-free, and we often compared notes on our health and diet. One day she mentioned very briefly that she had just taken a test that required her to drink a special solution and then blow into a tube every twenty minutes for three hours, and that, based on the results, she was now taking what she described as a radical antibiotic to try to solve her digestive problems. It turns out she'd taken the SIBO breath test, and her doctor had then determined she should take the antibiotic rifaximin (Xifaxan). Armed with this information, I called Dr. Run-Three-Miles for a prescription so that I could go to the University of South Florida and get tested myself (see page 16 for more on the SIBO breath test).

Three weeks after taking the test I received the results (these days you can get test results almost immediately and even take the test at home), which were negative. By that time, I had changed doctors and was seeing another gastroenterologist named Michael Schulman, who a friend had told me was a "digestion detective" and would definitely be able to help me. On my first visit, he sat with me for two hours, which to me was unbelievable, and he kept insisting that he wanted to see the full results from my test and interpret them himself. But I just kept saying that it had come back negative and shrugging it off. I was just too overwhelmed by everything I had to deal with to find that piece of paper or call the doctor's office to get it sent over. It took about a year and a half (really) before he finally convinced me to call my previous gastroenterologist's office. Part of my reluctance was undoubtedly because I'd already left the practice and therefore assumed that they'd give me a hard time. In the end, however, the woman who answered the phone couldn't have been nicer or more helpful.

When I handed the form to the "digestion detective," he told me that in fact I should have been told the test was positive—the results had been interpreted incorrectly. If I hadn't allowed my fear to hold me back, I could have had that information a lot sooner. I had learned my lesson.

So now I knew. Not only did I have IBS; I had the number one underlying cause of IBS, small intestine bacterial overgrowth (SIBO). Bacteria were overgrowing in my small intestine, causing my symptoms. That was a huge turning point for me. Finally, I not only had a name for my condition, I also had an explanation for symptoms that were terrorizing me. For the first time, I had hope that I might find a cure.

I wasn't alone, and I wondered how many other people were struggling with pain and had no idea it was being caused by SIBO. I was both angry and relieved. I vowed to find out everything I could about SIBO. The more research I did, the clearer it became that there wasn't very much information to be had from the usual mainstream sources. My life suddenly had an additional purpose—to become as much of an expert as possible and pass on my knowledge to as many people as would listen. I wanted to know everything: How many people have IBS? How many have SIBO? What percentage has only IBS and what percentage has both? How did I get it? What were the treatments? How could I keep myself from ever getting it again once I was cured? My starting point for fulfilling that purpose was to develop an increasingly intimate relationship with Dr. Google, meaning that I was on a DIY quest for information. That isn't unusual for people with problems about which the traditional medical community isn't necessarily well informed, but it can lead to information that is often controversial and can sometimes be misleading. It shouldn't, but often does, at least for a while, take the place of a doctor's visit. But the good news is that it also connects people to good doctors whom they would otherwise never have known about.

Eventually my exhaustive online searching led me to Dr. Allison Siebecker, a brilliant naturopathic physician who is a fellow SIBO sufferer and whose medical career is devoted to SIBO. Her website, siboinfo.com, has been an invaluable resource to millions of people and helped put SIBO on the map. When I reached out to her initially, she was concentrating on research and wasn't taking any new patients, so I continued to see my gastroenterologist. Thankfully, he was open to considering whatever information I was able to gather from my own research, and willing to try new treatments that had shown promise in trials or helped other patients. I would literally walk into his office with a study I'd printed off PubMed and he'd read it right there while I waited. He was smart, he was humble, and he was open to suggestions.

### Know Before You Go—to the Doctor

You've finally made an appointment to see a doctor, and whether you're using telemedicine or visiting someone the old-fashioned way, you really need to be prepared in order to maximize every moment with your expert of choice. Here are a few tips on what you need to know, what you need to take with you, and what you need to ask in order to make your doctor's appointment as efficient, informative, and effective as possible.

- Don't Depend on Your Memory. Trust me on this one. Make a list of what you want to cover and check it twice. I have walked out of the office more than once only to cuss loudly in the parking lot because of what I'd forgotten to ask! You can even audio record your conversations with your doctor so that you can review them again later. (Be sure to ask for permission first.)

- Know Your Symptoms. Write down all the symptoms you've been experiencing and when they occurred, even if you think they might not be relevant. Indicate any symptoms that are new. Include symptoms that come and go, too.

- Keep Track of Your History. Make a list of all tests you may already have taken, along with when they were done, and take copies of the results you were given. Tell your doctor what diagnoses you received from other doctors, and bring notes about treatments other practitioners tried and how you felt afterward.

- Discuss What You've Tried on Your Own. Have you been experimenting with treatments at home? What were the results?

- Bring Your Research. Make copies of any studies you have found to leave for your doctor to review.

- Determine What Tests You'd Like Your Doctor to Run and Why. This is where having a study to show the efficacy of the test could definitely be helpful.

- Decide What Prescriptions You Want the Doctor to Fill. Bring any written information or studies you have to show why they are effective. Write down your pharmacy information to leave with the doctor. If you are really anxious and afraid your pharmacy won't carry the medication you'll be asking for, call the pharmacy in advance to find out if they think they will have a hard time getting it quickly. I've done this on more than one occasion, and the pharmacist thanked me for giving him (or her) a heads-up.

- Be Nice! Thank the gatekeepers. Those overworked front desk folks are possibly the difference between getting your next appointment when you need it or waiting months and months. A smile and a thank-you go a long way. (Remembering their names is nice, too.)

- You Are the Customer. Remember, you have the power to fire your doctor if you are not feeling that you are getting the care you need.
- Keep a Question Journal. Keep a big list of all your questions in one place and, as they get answered by your research or your doctor, you can check them off. I find that doing that really gives me a sense of accomplishment and lets me feel that I'm making progress, even when things don't seem to be going so well.

AND YES, all this requires you to be super organized. It is a pain in the neck but worth it. I know.

Meanwhile, I stalked the appointment page of Dr. Siebecker's website on and off for a year until, one day, I saw that, miraculously, she was back from her research hiatus. I immediately booked ten appointments with her. I know this sounds crazy—in truth it seemed crazy to me at the time, especially since we were going to have to work together remotely. I wasn't yet familiar with telemedicine, but since I was able to send her my various test results and then describe my symptoms and reactions over Skype, it wasn't really necessary for me to be physically sitting in her exam room. Do keep this in mind as you search for your own doctor. You don't have to be constrained by geography—telemedicine is an extremely viable alternative, allowing you to see specialists no matter where they live. It is one of the best uses of the Internet I can think of—that and cat videos, of course.

Once we began working together, I started to get a better understanding of what SIBO actually was. I was surprised at every one of our sessions to learn something new—such as the fact that the herbs that helped one type of SIBO could make another type worse; what tests to take and in what order; and, yes, what to eat (and what not to eat!).

And throughout the process Dr. Siebecker assured me that among the complicated cases she usually saw, mine was not atypical. She believed that together we would get to the root of my problem, heal my intestines, and figure out how to manage my health going forward. But it was going to take time, and we might wind up having to take a few detours along the way. I was so relieved. My stress level was going down for the first time in years. We had a plan, and I was finally regaining my sense of hope.

At that point, my determination to be a patient advocate really kicked in. My husband was studying for his CPA exam, and for the first time since the '80s I had some time on my hands. I was on a mission— not only to heal myself but to use my story as well as the information I was gathering to prevent other people from having to go down the same long and painful road I had traveled. So, I started to keep a journal and make notes about what I learned. Typically, doctors are not taught much about SIBO in traditional medical schools—Dr. Siebecker has brought SIBO curriculum into naturopathic medical schools, but traditional medical schools do not offer training in it. So, as an educated patient, I knew I could become a desperately needed source on healing for both myself and for others. Before I knew it, I'd done so much research that I realized I could write an entire book.

Every medical practitioner I've worked with has encouraged me to share this information with others because they know firsthand how hard it is for SIBO sufferers to find advice they can trust. But it was really the encouragement of Linda Bennett, my spiritual teacher, that convinced me I must really sit down and write this book.

In this book, I've brought together all I have learned about SIBO over the years, including the plan that helped me get my life back.

## HOW TO USE THIS BOOK

In the following pages, I'll explain exactly what SIBO is, what causes it, and what puts you at risk. Then, we're going to dive into a plan that will help you feel 90 percent better in only 21 days and teach you how to resolve your SIBO for good. Here are the important steps:

### Step 1: Get Tested
Find out if SIBO is actually what ails you: You'll learn all about testing for SIBO in Chapter 1.

### Step 2: Learn Quick Symptom-Relief Strategies
Discover the tried-and-true tricks doctors and patients rely on to start feeling better right away. You'll find all this information in Chapter 3.

### Step 3: Remake Your Diet
In Chapters 4 and 5 you'll learn exactly what to eat and what to avoid to help reduce symptoms and feel better, including a 21-day meal plan with simple recipes.

### Step 4: Choose the Right Treatment
Diet alone won't get rid of SIBO, so in Chapter 6, I explain the medical treatments you can use to kick this condition for good.

### Step 5: Manage Your Symptoms over Time
In Chapter 7 you'll learn what to do moving forward to keep on feeling good.

The plan in this book will not only help you overcome SIBO but will also empower you with an understanding of what is happening in your body. You'll be more confident talking with your doctor, and if symptoms flare up, you'll understand why and what to do to get back to feeling better.

My journey with SIBO has been full of trial and error, but, ultimately, my life has been completely transformed, and yours can be, too. In this book, I'll distill what I've learned and offer you the powerful tools that will help you get your health back on track.

# CHAPTER 1

# What Is SIBO and How Do You Get It?

SIBO stands for small intestine bacterial overgrowth. It is a kind of microbial dysbiosis, or an imbalance in the small intestine. It is often confused with an infection, but it is not, as the overgrown bacteria aren't pathogenic in the traditional sense. The problem occurs when specific organisms overgrow in the small intestine. When they do, it creates a variety of health challenges. SIBO is a condition caused by something else, and it causes symptoms of its own.

Most people have never heard of SIBO, much less know what those letters stand for. I've been interested in health for as long as I can remember, so I couldn't believe I had never heard of SIBO. That is the exact reason why I wrote this book: to help shine a light on a health issue that has not gotten enough attention.

What actually happens in your body after you chew your food and before you poop remains something of a mystery for most of us. So, before you can understand SIBO, you really need to know a little bit more about digestion.

When you chew and swallow food, it goes down your esophagus and into your stomach first. Your stomach actually sits much higher in your abdomen than you might think—right underneath your rib cage. The food is broken down by stomach acid (which also helps kill any pathogens or bacteria that traveled in on your food). Then, from the stomach, chyme, which is food that's now partially digested and mixed with stomach acid, moves into the small intestine.

At just about twenty feet long, the small intestine is actually longer than your large intestine. It sits coiled in your lower belly with the large intestine wrapped around it. In the small intestine, chyme is broken down into nutrients that can be absorbed by your body, which then move down to your large intestine, where the vast majority of bacteria are supposed to live.

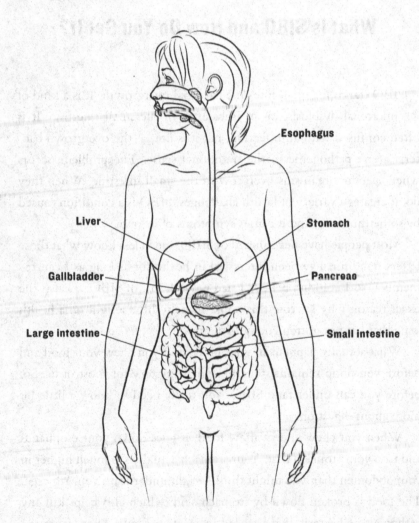

The trillions of bacteria and other microorganisms in your large intestine are collectively known as your intestinal microbiome. In total, they weigh about the same amount as your brain and help perform many necessary functions. In addition to occupying your large intestine, bacteria also live in your mouth, on your skin, and even in your genitals, all of which have their own microbiomes.

Normally, your small intestine should contain very few bacteria. Many are killed by stomach acid before they even reach the small intestine; others are quickly flushed out and moved into the large intestine. But under certain conditions bacteria begin to proliferate in the small intestine and then feed on particular kinds of carbohydrates you have eaten. The bacteria turn these carbohydrates into acids and gas. The medical term for that process is fermentation.

Some of the specific bacteria found in research to overgrow and cause SIBO include Christensenellaceae, Ruminococcaceae, Fusobacterium, and Desulfovibrio. But don't panic, you don't need to remember these names, what is important is the type of gas the bacteria create: hydrogen, hydrogen sulfide, or methane. And because the bacteria are in the small intestine, the gas then causes a whole confluence of symptoms that range from mildly embarrassing to seriously painful and debilitating, including bloating, cramps, nausea, acid reflux, diarrhea, constipation, and more. (Methane is associated with constipation, hydrogen is associated with diarrhea, and hydrogen sulfide is associated with diarrhea.)

SIBO is like real estate—it's all about location, location, location.

The fermentation of carbohydrates in the small intestine can even lead to either weight loss or weight gain with malnutrition, because the bacteria interfere with proper digestion and either increase the number of calories your body absorbs or use up vital nutrients to feed themselves instead of feeding you. And that, in a nutshell, is small intestine bacterial overgrowth.

If you've noticed that the symptoms of SIBO are basically the same as those used to describe and define irritable bowel syndrome (IBS), that's because SIBO is often the cause of IBS. Recent data suggest that up to 78 percent of people with IBS have SIBO. The problem is that most people never get past treating their symptoms to finding, and addressing, the root cause.

## IBS, SIBO, and IBD

IBS is irritable bowel syndrome; IBD is inflammatory bowel disease. It's important to know the difference between the two and to understand how SIBO came to be stuck in the middle. Irritable bowel syndrome is basically diagnosed based on a collection of symptoms including abdominal pain or discomfort, diarrhea or constipation or both, and bloating that have no other obvious cause. You probably wouldn't be diagnosed with IBS until other causes of your symptoms had been ruled out. But, in the majority of cases, those symptoms are caused by SIBO, which is the one thing for which you probably won't be tested. Now you can see why so many people live with this condition for so long.

Inflammatory bowel disease, on the other hand, is a serious condition that includes ulcerative colitis, which is defined by inflammation of the colon, and Crohn's disease, in which the inflammation affects the entire GI tract. Therefore, if you have digestive symptoms, it's very important to rule out IBD before assuming it is "just" IBS or SIBO.

At the same time, it's important to note that both Crohn's and colitis can cause SIBO via structural changes.

So, to be clear, SIBO can (and most often does) cause IBS, and IBD (that is, Crohn's disease or colitis) can cause SIBO.

As I've said, many doctors still don't know much, if anything, about SIBO, so IBS is generally accepted as a final diagnosis rather than a group of symptoms requiring further investigation. Therefore, while it's sometimes frowned upon for patients to take control of their health by consulting Dr. Google, in the case of SIBO it really is essential that you do so. Although it is just now becoming better understood, many doctors still have never heard of SIBO, let alone know what tests are needed to diagnose it or the multistep treatment protocols that can eradicate it.

And if you feel silly or embarrassed bringing this information to your doctor, I understand. It can be intimidating to tell a doctor, "I think I have this." But many physicians have actually thanked me for the work I'm doing to educate their patients, since there is so little awareness of SIBO in either medical or popular health circles.

In fact, if you have IBS and you've come across this book, this may very well be your lucky day. Millions of people with IBS believe that all they can do to deal with their situation is to be very careful about what they eat and take laxatives or antidiarrheals for the rest of their life—which is, of course, the very definition of treating the symptoms instead of the disease.

For a long time, that was me, but now I know better. There is help. There is hope, and answers do exist. Not only can you start to feel better quite quickly, but there is also hope for a drastic reduction of symptoms, remission, and, yes, in many cases a cure.

But if SIBO can cause IBS, that begs the question: What causes SIBO? The small intestine normally has many protections against bacterial accumulation. They are:

- stomach acid, which kills bacteria
- bile, which also kills bacteria
- enzymes, which kill bacteria or arrest their growth
- the immune system, which kills bacteria and all kinds of other invaders
- normal small intestine anatomy, which moves the bacteria through and out of the small intestine

- the ileocecal valve, which is designed to prevent bacteria from the large intestine from backing up into the small intestine
- the migrating motor complex, which moves bacteria out of the small intestine

I'll be explaining all of these in detail in the pages that follow, but for the moment, I want you to understand that, according to Dr. Siebecker, one or more of these protections needs to fail in order for SIBO to occur. And remember, it's not a question of whether the bacteria are good or bad, or how they overgrew in the small intestine in the first place. We know that bacteria either sneak down from above, overgrow from within the small intestine, or move back up from the large intestine below. It's really about having too many bacteria in the wrong place.

So now we have to wonder, why would one or more of these protections fail? We need to think about why the bacteria aren't being removed. Why are they not being handled? Why are they accumulating? What was the underlying cause of your SIBO?

**By far the most common cause of SIBO is food poisoning.** Approximately one in six Americans or forty-eight million people (and one in ten or about eight hundred million worldwide) get a foodborne illness every year, and approximately 10 percent of them will then develop "postinfectious" IBS, which in this case is caused by SIBO. According to the newest research, IBS caused by food poisoning is SIBO. In fact, Dr. Mark Pimentel, an internationally known SIBO researcher and executive director of the Medically Associated Science and Technology (MAST) Program at Cedars-Sinai Medical Center, believes that "about 60 to 70 percent of IBS is caused by food poisoning, especially IBS with diarrhea." The MAST Program focuses on the development of drugs, diagnostic tests, and devices related to conditions of the microbiome.

## FOOD POISONING AND SIBO—A POTENTIALLY VICIOUS CYCLE

I'm sure you've heard about foods being recalled because they might contain E. coli or salmonella, *Campylobacter jejuni*, or shigella. What you might not realize, however, is that those are all types of bacteria that produce a nerve toxin called cytolethal distending toxin B (Cdt-B), which causes acute gastroenteritis—commonly known as food poisoning. When we get food poisoning our body produces antibodies to fight and destroy the bacteria and their toxins, and for about 90 percent of us that means we first suffer a severe bout of diarrhea or vomiting (or both), and then the army of antibodies that's been deployed to fight the bacteria does its job, they go back to their barracks, we get better, and that's that. But for the remaining 10 percent, it could well mean the onset of SIBO. If you think 10 percent sounds like a relatively low number, remember that about forty-eight million Americans get food poisoning every year. Ten percent of forty-eight million is almost five million people who could potentially get SIBO every year in the United States alone.

Here's why: When you're exposed to Cdt-B toxin because you have food poisoning, the antibodies you produce to fight it can get confused and, in effect, start a war with the wrong adversary. This happens because parts of the Cdt-B toxin are very similar in structure to vinculin, a protein that plays a key role in connecting nerve cells to one another. So, sometimes the antibodies designed to bind with and fight-off the Cdt-B toxin mistakenly bind with vinculin as well, killing off a key protein in your body with friendly fire—or, in more scientific terms, you experience an autoimmune response. We know this because, after a bout of food poisoning, blood tests might show that you have antibodies to both Cdt-B and vinculin.

Digestion itself takes place in the small intestine (which is about twenty feet long, four times longer than the large intestine), and the waste products of the digestive process then move down through the large intestine and are ultimately excreted in your stool. When the vinculin is compromised, it damages the nerves that help create the migrating motor complex (MMC), a type of peristalsis that sweeps through your intestines after you've finished digesting and moves any leftover particles from your small intestine into your large intestine and, eventually, out of your body through elimination. It's often called the "housekeeper wave" and I think of it like someone coming through and sweeping all the crumbs out of your small intestine and into your large intestine.

Have you ever been sitting in a meeting only to be mortified by the sound of your stomach grumbling? That grumble sound is actually created by your migrating motor complex at work. It's nothing to be embarrassed about; in fact, it's actually a sign that your body is doing what it is supposed to do. In a healthy person, the migrating motor complex should be "turned on" between meals and occur at ninety-minute intervals so long as you've finished digesting and haven't eaten anything since.

When the MMC is compromised, that sweeping doesn't take place enough, so the bacteria remain in your small intestine and start to overgrow, "eating" whatever undigested food is there, fermenting it into gas, which in turn creates bloating and other symptoms. Bottom line: You get SIBO/IBS. In fact, the number one physiologic underlying cause of SIBO is thought to be slow motility in the small intestine—that is, a deficient migrating motor complex, most often caused by food poisoning.

Don't remember having food poisoning? If not, you may still have had a mild case. But even a mild case of food poisoning can trigger IBS. And even if you haven't been diagnosed with food poisoning, if you've had a bout of diarrhea or thought you had the stomach flu, you may very well have had food poisoning. Since the symptoms are the same, it's hard to tell them apart. Unless you got tested at the time, you wouldn't know if it was bacterial or viral. It's the bacterial food poisoning that leads to SIBO/IBS.

Some people might have acute food poisoning and then they get better but continue to have some diarrhea because now they have SIBO. But for others, SIBO onset can be delayed for up to three months, which makes it difficult to connect that bout of food poisoning with the onset of SIBO. Of course, not everyone who gets food poisoning goes on to develop SIBO, but just having this information could help make you more vigilant about what you're eating, where it comes from, and the long-term effects it might have.

Plus, if you have SIBO from food poisoning (postinfectious IBS), you're more likely to get food poisoning again. You could sit at the same table and eat the same food as others, and be the only one who gets sick, because your MMC has already been compromised. You might think that people who travel a lot—particularly to countries whose sanitation systems are different from ours—would be the ones at risk, but simply eating at your local salad bar might also put you at risk.

That's why I encourage anyone with digestive issues like IBS or SIBO to be tested for anti–Cdt-B and anti–vinculin antibodies. It's a simple blood test called ibs-smart that can reveal a lot about your health, but it's also relatively new, so you'll probably have to ask your doctor to order it for you, and you may even have to inform him or her that it exists.

If your blood tests positive, as mine did, there's a more than 95 percent chance that your SIBO/IBS was caused by food poisoning (which is also known as "postinfectious IBS"). I know that I previously said IBS was a functional disorder diagnosed only by a process of elimination, but this new test is changing that. Just knowing that you have postinfectious IBS (SIBO from food poisoning) can tell you a lot about what treatments might work best for you and what you can do to avoid getting it again.

## ADHESIONS AND OTHER OBSTRUCTIONS

Adhesions are basically internal scars made of collagen fibers, and for the most part they serve a useful purpose by holding things together after a trauma such as surgery or even something as ordinary as falling off your bicycle or getting hit in the stomach with a ball as a kid. Mine came from having a seat belt dig into me when I was in a car accident. But what makes adhesions so powerful can make them so difficult to live with because the collagen fibers of which they are made are pound-for-pound stronger than steel. Think about a heavy-duty rope tied in knots so tight there's nothing you can do to unknot them. That's a good way to envision an adhesion. And sometimes, depending on where they are in your body, adhesions can physically obstruct the normal flow of the small intestine and prevent bacteria from moving through as they should.

Ironically (and unfortunately), very often, when people develop adhesions following surgery, the response of traditional medicine is to do another surgery to remove them, which may then lead to even more adhesions. Not unlike repeated cases of food poisoning, repeated surgeries can create a vicious cycle that increases your risk for developing SIBO.

A little known fact is that endometriosis is another cause of adhesions and, therefore, a cause of SIBO. When endometrial tissue grows outside the uterus, that buildup of tissue can cause inflammation, which then leads to the formation of scar tissue. Ironically, scar tissue is part of the healing process.

## Treating Adhesions

For years surgery was the only treatment option, but now there's a new technique that was pioneered by Larry Wurn, LMT, the founder and director of Clear Passage, a network of research and treatment clinics in the United States and the United Kingdom that treat adhesion-related problems, including bowel obstructions, SIBO, and pain. The Wurn Technique is a hands-on,

> noninvasive treatment that can dissolve adhesions. Find a
> Wurn practitioner at http://www.clearpassage.com/who-we-are
> /locations/.
>
> Visceral manipulation is another hands-on technique that has
> been very beneficial for me with adhesions. Find a visceral
> manipulation practitioner at https://www.barralinstitute.com/.
>
> Another form of relatively noninvasive treatment is neural
> therapy, which involves injecting a kind of Novocain into a
> specific area.

In addition to adhesions, there are structural problems that can cause SIBO, such as small intestine diverticulosis, which means that you have pockets protruding from the wall of your small intestinal tract because the SIBO bacteria tend to accumulate in those pockets.

Your small intestine is quite literally like a hose, and we all know what happens to a hose with a twist or a kink in it: Water backs up. You can be born with a twist or kink in your intestines (so think back to how long you've had digestive issues), but you can also develop one as a result of surgery, or it can happen later in life. Stricture, compression, or even a tumor in the small intestine (to name just a few), could also physically obstruct and prevent the clearance of the microbes, leading to SIBO.

And then there's blind loop syndrome, which occurs when a segment of the small intestine gets cut off from the flow of the MMC from a certain type of surgery, creating the perfect conditions for bacteria to start multiplying.

Since blind loop syndrome, kinks, twists, strictures, and adhesions can all result from abdominal or intestinal surgery of any kind, if you've ever had an appendectomy, a C-section, a gastric bypass, or any other type of abdominal surgery, these possible causes of SIBO should definitely be on your radar.

## PROKINETICS—WHAT THEY ARE AND WHAT THEY DO

Prokinetics are a group of drugs that work to keep food and bacteria moving through your digestive tract. Slowed small intestine motility is one of the most common causes of SIBO.

Multiple factors can affect motility, but food poisoning may be the most common. Food poisoning that causes postinfectious IBS slows small intestine motility because the autoimmune response attacks the vinculin, which then causes your migrating motor complex to stop functioning as it should. If you have postinfectious IBS from food poisoning, you'll want to be sure that you're taking prokinetics to help get things moving.

Prokinetics are not laxatives; their purpose is to stimulate the MMC so that the bacteria are swept out of your small intestine instead of building up where they don't belong. Depending on the dose, they may or may not cause you to have a bowel movement. Doses of prokinetics for those with SIBO are low and can be taken by those with diarrhea.

An important note: Prokinetics should always be taken on an empty stomach so that they can stimulate the MMC. Personally, I take mine at night, since I know I'll be fasting while I'm asleep.

### Dr. Siebecker's Recommended Prokinetics

#### PRESCRIPTION

Low-dose prucalopride (0.5–I mg per day), sold in the United States under the brand name Motegrity (called Resolor or Resotran in other countries).

Low-dose erythromycin (50 mg per day). It isn't sold in such a low dose unless you have it specially compounded, but you can ask your doctor to prescribe a 250-mg pill and cut it in quarters with a pill cutter.

Low-dose naltrexone (LDN for short) (2.5–5 mg per day). This is generally used in combination with other prokinetics and has many benefits, including reducing inflammation, helping autoimmunity, and reducing pain. Dosing varies, so work with a practitioner. This medication literally changed my life. Find out more at https://ldnresearchtrust.org/.

**HERBAL/NATURAL**

Iberogast (see page 47)

Ginger Root. There have been many studies on the use of ginger as a prokinetic. Many people swear by it, but it can cause "ginger burn" in some people, which is a hot feeling in the esophagus. If you have acid reflux, this would probably not be a good choice for you.

Dr. Siebecker recommends the following prokinetics that contain ginger, as well:

- Prokine (Vita Aid)
- MotilPro (Pure Encapsulations)
- Motility Activator (Integrative Therapeutics)
- GI Motility Complex (Enzyme Science)
- SIBO-MMC (Priority One)
- Bio.Me Kinetic (Invivo, UK)

I should also mention here that if your SIBO was, in fact, caused by food poisoning, you may need to remain on low doses of prescription or herbal prokinetics for life and/or rotate them to keep your symptoms at bay.

## MEDICATIONS—A DOUBLE-EDGED SWORD?

It's unfortunate but true that the very medications you take to save your life can also have unintended life-altering side effects, one of which might be developing SIBO.

Antibiotic use can lead to SIBO by slowing intestinal motility. This is confusing for many because antibiotics are also used to treat SIBO. But the antibiotics used for SIBO are very specific and uniquely suited to treat SIBO. I'll explain exactly why and how in the coming chapters.

According to a primary care review published in the December 2016 *Mayo Clinic Proceedings,* patients who use narcotics—and opioids in particular—or proton-pump inhibitors are at increased risk for developing SIBO.

Opioids are generally prescribed for pain management, and while they may be effective for reducing pain in both the short and the long term, they also are known for causing opioid-induced bowel dysfunction whose symptoms include constipation, anorexia, nausea, vomiting, gastroesophageal reflux disease (heartburn or GERD), delayed digestion, abdominal pain, flatulence, bloating, hard stool, straining during bowel movement, and incomplete evacuation. In general, they slow things down, including digestion and, particularly, the functioning of the MMC, so it's no coincidence that many of these symptoms are the same as the symptoms of SIBO.

When you're given anesthesia for surgery, digestion is suppressed, and then, after surgery, you're given opioids for pain. In effect, you're being hit with a double whammy. But even people who take opioids in the short term to treat pain from an acute condition such as shingles or even a dental procedure very often find their digestion is disrupted. Dr. Mark Pimentel has told me that as little as a few days of opioids can lead to SIBO if the MMC is already compromised, so using a prokinetic anytime you take opioids is important for prevention.

## RADIATION

At least one study has found that 20 to 25 percent of people who receive pelvic radiation develop gastrointestinal problems associated with SIBO. My friend Karen was one of those people who developed SIBO after receiving radiation after cancer surgery, which also left her with adhesions.

Intestinal radiation toxicity, also called post-radiation enteropathy, can cause a wide range of symptoms (including pain after eating, obstruction of the small intestine, bloating, diarrhea, and the inability to absorb various nutrients) that may be caused by damage done to the small intestine itself, by bacterial overgrowth, or by lactose intolerance—all of which are associated with SIBO.

## THYROID ISSUES

The thyroid is a butterfly-shaped gland located in the neck that produces hormones. It is closely linked to the gut, and even formed at the same time as the gut in utero. Thyroid issues, both hyper- and hypothyroidism, and SIBO can have the same symptoms: weight gain or loss, constipation, diarrhea, bloating, and fatigue. However, thyroid issues can also be an underlying cause for SIBO, as the hormones produced by the thyroid can impact motility directly, with hypothyroidism causing constipation.

## WHY KNOWING THE CAUSE IS IMPORTANT

As you can see, it's complicated, and sometimes getting to the root cause can be like trying to solve a really knotty problem. In fact, you might be wondering why that even matters. "I have this thing and I want to get rid of it. Why does it matter how I got it?" The answer is that the cause may, at least to some degree, dictate the cure.

In addition, it's essential to determine the cause of your symptoms because SIBO can present with the same symptoms as other diseases, so you can't really be sure you have it unless you take the SIBO breath test.

## THE SIBO BREATH TEST

The best way to determine if you have SIBO is to take the SIBO breath test. Most breath tests check for the presence of hydrogen and methane, two gases created by the SIBO-producing organisms. As of this writing, a new test can also determine the presence of hydrogen sulfide gas, as well as hydrogen and methane. This is important because it is one of the factors that determines what type of SIBO you have and, therefore, what type of treatment will work best for you. Methane is associated with constipation, while hydrogen and hydrogen sulfide are associated with diarrhea. Research has also shown that as PPM (parts per million) of hydrogen sulfide rises, so does diarrhea severity.

Why a breath test instead of an MRI, an X-ray, or a CT scan? Because the SIBO overgrowth doesn't show up on that kind of imaging. You may have heard or been told that you can take a stool test or a urine organic acid test, but neither one of those really works for diagnosing SIBO. The stool test actually reflects what is in the *large* intestine, and the urine test can show that there is a bacterial overgrowth somewhere in the large or small intestine, but it doesn't show *which location specifically* has the overgrowth. A small bowel culture could theoretically diagnose SIBO, but because the small intestine is so long, and so deeply nestled inside your body, doing any sort of test like that is very invasive. And even then, these tests can't reach much past the first few inches of the small intestine and, therefore, might not detect SIBO farther along, even when it is present.

Endoscopy will show the upper portion of the (not so small) small intestine, and a colonoscopy will show the lower portion, but the approximately seventeen feet in the middle are not shown in either of these tests, according to Dr. Siebecker.

That doesn't mean that these tests might not be useful for determining whether you have a problem other than SIBO or that is also causing SIBO. You should discuss their potential efficacy with your doctor, but the bottom line is that if you suspect SIBO, the best way to rule it out (or in) is with a breath test, and there is no reason why you shouldn't be able to take one.

## Taking the SIBO Breath Test

Before you take the test you'll need to do a bit of advance planning. To prepare, you need to follow a very restricted diet for twelve hours and then fast overnight for twelve hours before taking the test. The only foods allowed for vegetarians on the prep diet are eggs, sometimes potatoes, sometimes cheese, white rice, white bread, black coffee or tea with no dairy or sweetener, and water. If it isn't on the list, you can't have it, so be sure to check the specific diet that comes with your test. I know, it sounds terrible, even for those of you who may have already been following a restricted diet for SIBO. But it's for a good reason: The point is to lower your carbohydrate levels so that the bacteria have nothing to feed on and you can, therefore, get a baseline gas level at the start of the test and see the bacterial response to the test solution. If you haven't properly completed the prep, you won't get accurate results, so don't cheat! If you have constipation, you might be better off following the prep diet for two days to be sure you get accurate results.

Once you've completed the prep, you drink a particular kind of sugar solution (glucose or lactulose, as discussed below) that feeds the bacteria and thus encourages them to produce gas. The presence and quantity of the bacteria are determined by the amount of gas produced, because humans do not normally produce these gases, which are by-products of the fermentation of carbohydrates consumed by the bacteria.

It takes some advance prep and it is time-consuming but is otherwise painless.

## Lactulose versus Glucose

There are two types of sugar solution that can be used in the SIBO breath test.

**Glucose** is available without a prescription but is of limited value because it only tests for SIBO bacteria that are in the first two or three feet of the small intestine (your small intestine can be seventeen to twenty-five-feet long). So, you might get a false negative result.

**Lactulose** is a different type of sugar solution that, in the United States, can be obtained only with a prescription but is more likely to provide an accurate result because it tests all the way down to the bottom of the small intestine and because humans cannot digest or absorb lactulose; only bacteria have the enzyme that allows them to do this.

When the bacteria "eat" the lactulose they make hydrogen and methane gas, particularly in the small intestine, which then enters your bloodstream and travels to the lungs, where it is released when you breathe. Hence, the SIBO "breath" test.

You then blow into a tube every twenty minutes over the course of three hours to capture that gas. It generally takes about two hours for the lactulose to travel through the small intestine, but if you have a slow transit time (which I do), it may take longer; therefore, doing the three hours provides a safety net, so to speak, even though some doctors will tell you it isn't necessary. According to Dr. Siebecker, a three-hour test also represents methane and hydrogen sulfide better than a shorter test.

Humans can't make methane or hydrogen gas on their own, so if they are present in high amounts in the small intestine, it means you have SIBO. But reading the results isn't as black and white as it might seem, so it's important that you see a doctor who is familiar with SIBO and with what the test results really mean. When my "digestive detective" doctor reread the results of my SIBO breath test, he saw that they clearly showed a spike in hydrogen in my body, indicating the presence of bacteria. My first doctor had completely missed this.

My personal experience with this test is that the lactulose didn't make me feel very well, probably because of all the fermentation it created, and I also didn't enjoy sitting in the doctor's waiting room for three hours, periodically breathing into a tube. For those reasons I much prefer to take the test at home, which many doctors will let you do. In fact, there's even a kit you can use to collect your breath samples at home and then mail them to a lab to be tested. Whether you do it at home or in a doctor's office, however, my advice is to be your own "digestion detective" and get as much information as you can. Get the test results printed out and look at the graph yourself.

One caveat is that simply taking the test can create—or increase—SIBO-induced brain fog (see page 32), so you need to be very careful (or have someone help you) with labeling the samples. I once had to scrap an entire test—after doing the prep and completing almost the entire three hours—because I spaced out on the labeling near the end. For that reason, I recommend that you use two timers—a kitchen-type timer and one on your phone. Trust me on this. It isn't worth getting confused and forgetting something that causes you to go through the whole thing all over again. And label everything before you start.

It also makes sense to do the test first thing in the morning, since you have to fast for twelve hours before taking it, and, based on my own experience, I would suggest giving yourself the rest of the day off. Don't make any big plans for what to do afterward. Some people do just fine, even taking the test at work in between meetings! But for me, creating all that gas caused my symptoms to flare up, and all I wanted to do was lie down and rest as soon as possible. In addition to the simple stress of completing the test, restricting your carb intake and then drinking a sugar solution can really mess with your blood sugar levels, as it definitely did with mine.

You can order the test yourself, your doctor can give you a prescription to order the test, or they can order it for you to take either at home or in the office. Having said that, it's possible that your doctor won't be familiar with the test or won't want to order it. You'd be amazed by how often that happens. So, my advice is to take all of your information with you. Not even the most knowledgeable doctors can know everything about everything, but they should at least be open to learning. That said, even if your doctor is open-minded, if he or she isn't familiar with the breath test, it might be time for you to look for a new doctor who is. If someone doesn't know the test, there's a good chance he also won't know how to interpret the results or which treatments would be appropriate.

### How and Where to Get the Lactulose Breath Test

In case your doctor isn't familiar with the SIBO breath test or doesn't know how to order it, here are some of the facilities offering the test in the United States.* Some will ship the test to you directly.

Aerodiagnostics: 844-681-9449

Breath Trackers/QuinTron (hydrogen sulfide testing available in 2021): 800-542-4448

SIBO Center Lab, National University of Natural Medicine (NUNM): 503-552-1931

Trio Smart Breath Test (tests for all three gases: hydrogen sulfide, methane, and hydrogen): https://www.triosmartbreathtest.com/

*For the most up-to-date information on how and where to get the test, please see https://www.sibointo.com/testing.html.

## Why Testing Is Important

Taking the breath test can seem like a lot of work, and you might be tempted to skip it entirely. But knowing for certain that you have SIBO, and what type you have, is a huge step forward in the healing process. And because the symptoms of SIBO are so general and can be caused by many conditions, it's important to be sure what you're dealing with so that you don't overlook something else.

Doctors often make a diagnosis based on symptoms alone, but Dr. Siebecker taught me that there are thirty-five to forty other diseases that could cause the very same symptoms as SIBO but would require very different treatment. Lactose intolerance, for example, may cause the same symptoms, but the treatment is taking lactase enzymes. There have been studies examining how well you can diagnose SIBO based on symptoms, and the answer is not well at all. One study compared the symptoms reported by people with small intestine fungal over-growth (SIFO) to those reported by people who had SIBO, and what they found was that the reported symptoms were indistinguishable. Since the most accurate test for SIFO is to do an endoscopy, which requires sedation, it would make sense to test for SIBO first and avoid the more invasive test if possible.

In addition to SIFO, however, SIBO can also mimic parasites or something far more serious that needs to be dealt with as quickly as possible. So if you don't get to the bottom of what's bothering you, you could be wasting your time treating the wrong illness or, worse, allowing what your real problem is to progress even more.

### Parasites and SIBO

No one likes talking about it, but the fact is that parasites exist, and most people have them. They're everywhere—in our food, in our water supply, in salad bars—and they don't recognize borders, according to naturopathic physician Dr. Anne Hill. But the good news is that they don't always make you sick because your immune system may fight them off. That said, if you're having gastrointestinal problems and you don't know why, it would be a good idea to get tested for parasites. You may also be totally asymptomatic but still have a parasite, so testing is always a good idea.

**Parasite Warning Signs To Look Out For**
- Fatigue and insomnia
- Weight gain or loss
- Diarrhea or constipation
- Bloating
- Food sensitivities
- Have pets
- Work in garden/outdoors
- Past food poisoning
- Drink tap or well water
- Swimmer (pools, lakes, ocean, etc.)

The standard test for parasites is the O&P (ova and parasites) stool test, which is notorious for giving false negative results. So, don't be fooled! Most labs don't send their samples to a parasitologist; they just look at them on a slide, and they often don't know what they're looking for. Dr. Raphael d'Angelo at ParaWellness Research in Aurora, Colorado, is a parasitologist who can often find things other labs don't. You can order a test kit, send your specimen to his lab, and receive results along with treatment recommendations. Another good test for parasites is the comprehensive stool test GI-MAP.

If you've tested positive for SIBO and you have been treated but it keeps coming back, you could also have parasites, according to Dr. Ilana Gurevich. They can compete with the bacteria (and with you) for nourishment because they want to survive. In addition to stealing your food, however, parasites also work to shut down your immune system (another of their survival mechanisms), so, among other things, you might find that a food you did fine with last week triggers a reaction in you this week. In short, if you have SIBO and parasites, it may be virtually impossible to cure your SIBO until you've cleared out the parasites.

Different types of parasites require different treatment, which is why testing, retesting, and working with a knowledgeable practitioner are so important.

I absolutely urge you to do the detective work needed to find your underlying cause or causes. Remember that SIBO is a condition caused by something else, and if you don't know what that something else is, it is likely only a matter of time until your SIBO relapses. What if you can't figure out your underlying cause? It doesn't mean you'll never get better. You can still manage SIBO. However, with some digging and persistence, you just might be able to unravel the thread of what is causing your SIBO. I now know my SIBO was caused by food poisoning and postinfectious IBS.

With the help of some wonderful doctors and some powerful lifestyle changes, my symptoms are under control.

To view the references cited in this chapter, please visit healingsibo.com/references.

# CHAPTER 2

# Is SIBO Controlling My Weight and Making Me Anxious?

Let's do a quick review. The gas in SIBO is caused by bacteria in the small intestine consuming carbohydrates and fermenting them into gas. Different bacteria produce different gas: hydrogen, methane, or hydrogen sulfide. The different gases are associated with different symptoms. Hydrogen and hydrogen sulfide both tend to cause diarrhea and methane is associated with constipation. But methane gas sometimes has another side effect: weight gain. Studies suggest that methane can also make you feel anxious and depressed.

## IS SIBO AFFECTING MY WEIGHT?

### Methane and Weight Gain

Let me explain how methane can contribute to weight gain. The primary producers of methane are *Methanobrevibacter smithii*, which are extremely efficient in breaking down the food you eat and turning it into calories for your body to absorb and use as fuel. When you have a normal quantity of the bacteria, they will perform this function correctly, but when there's an overgrowth, your body will absorb more calories than it needs, and you may gain weight. This means that even if you consume the same foods in the same amounts as someone who does not have an *M. smithii* overgrowth, you will absorb more calories. Have you ever wondered why your girlfriend who eats exactly the same things you do is three pant sizes smaller? Methane could be a reason.

Methane, in effect, slows down the large and small intestine so that once the bacteria break down the foods you eat, you'll have a longer time to absorb the calories that are there. I know, because I've experienced it myself, and I can tell you that it was extremely frustrating, or, actually, quite maddening. And I'm not just talking about bloating, which is a whole different issue. My weight gain might not have been noticeable to anyone who didn't know me well, but I could feel the difference. All of a sudden, even though I was eating and exercising exactly the way I always had, nothing I'd been doing to maintain my weight was working for me anymore. My clothes didn't fit, and I didn't feel comfortable in my own body, which made me feel completely out of control.

Dr. Pimentel and his group have shown that in an obese population of people whose body mass index (BMI) was over thirty, those with methane dominant SIBO had a BMI that was seven points higher than those who didn't have methane. In addition, among the general population, those who had both methane and hydrogen on their breath test had a higher BMI than those who had hydrogen alone. While he hastens to add that these studies do not show cause and effect, they do show a positive association between methane and being overweight. I'm excited and hopeful for what this research could reveal in the future.

In a follow-up study, Dr. Ruchi Mathur, who is a member of Pimentel's group at Cedars-Sinai Hospital in Los Angeles, is currently looking at the effects that the content of your gut microbiome can have on the development of obesity and insulin resistance.

## Is *M. smithii* Overgrowth Really SIBO?

In a paper just published as I am writing this book, Dr. Mark Pimentel of Cedars-Sinai Medical Center proposes that because *M. smithii* are not actually bacteria but rather archaea, another type of organism that lives in the digestive tract, and because these archaea may overgrow in the colon as well as the small intestine, SIBO with constipation should not be called SIBO at all but rather IMO (intestinal methane overgrowth). The problem, he says, is "one of nomenclature. Excessive methane production cannot be caused by 'bacterial' overgrowth, but is rather due to archaeal overgrowth. Therefore, SIBO with methane should not be called SIBO at all, but rather IMO (Intestinal Methane Overgrowth)."

For the moment, however, the medical world has not caught up with Dr. Pimentel. So, rather than causing further confusion, I will continue to refer to SIBO with constipation or methane dominant SIBO in this book.

## SIBO CAN ALSO KEEP YOU MALNOURISHED

According to Dr. Siebecker, there are a lot of reasons for weight loss if you have SIBO, starting with the fact that if you're avoiding fermentable foods to manage your SIBO symptoms, you're automatically going to be on a low-carbohydrate diet and, therefore, you might see the number on the scale going down even if you aren't trying to lose weight. In addition, the small intestine is normally where food is broken down into absorbable nutrients, but, if you have SIBO, the bacteria may be stealing your food in order to feed themselves. Or, if you have a lot of diarrhea, that, too, can cause weight loss because the food is moving so quickly through the digestive system that there isn't time for it to be properly absorbed. And if one of your symptoms is that you're nauseated all the time, you probably won't want to eat very much to begin with. And, of course, being bloated and having belly pain can really cut down on your appetite.

To make matters worse, when people are really busy, they may skip a meal or two, so they don't experience a flare-up of symptoms. I know that when I did that, when I finally got home, I'd overeat because I was so hungry, and that, of course, would make me feel even worse.

It's a problem when something as basic as eating, which used to give you pleasure, is no longer pleasant because of the aftermath. When that happens, you need to make sure that you don't fall into unhealthy habits to provide satisfaction, such as excessive shopping, smoking, reckless gambling, and all of the other potential potholes. The struggle is real.

For a while I was so consumed with my own weight gain that I didn't really consider what it would be like for someone at the other end of the spectrum. It wasn't until a member of the SIBO SOS community told me about her own problems that I really began to understand what it would feel like to be too thin. She said she was devastated and, at one point, she actually thought she was going to die. Her entire family was worried about her, and everyone simply seemed to assume that she had an eating disorder. Losing weight as a result of SIBO can have serious, even life-threatening, consequences physically, emotionally, and psychologically.

## IS SIBO AFFECTING MY BRAIN?

Being sick wears you down; it's stressful and depressing—especially if, like so many people with SIBO, your problems are being misdiagnosed or misunderstood by your doctor.

If food makes you feel sick, you may start to avoid events where food is being served. Sometimes simply being around food you know you can't eat without feeling awful sucks the joy out of social events. Explaining why you eat the way you do, or why you're always in the bathroom, can make social situations awkward. And if you're trying to date or make new friends while struggling with SIBO, I know what that feels like. These are all very real and legitimate feelings. But once again, when you're dealing with SIBO there is much more to it than that. SIBO also affects hormones, which in turn influence both mental and gastrointestinal functions.

There are two modes within your nervous system: the sympathetic and the parasympathetic. In the simplest of terms, the sympathetic mode is fight or flight, and the parasympathetic is rest and digest. (If you have trouble remembering which is which, as I did, it might help to think of it this way: When you're stressed, you need sympathy.) SIBO and IBS can definitely make you feel more stressed, anxious, and depressed, feelings that lead to your body's increasing its production of cortisol, commonly called the "stress hormone." When cortisol is elevated, the digestive system effectively "shuts off" so that you can direct all of your energy to warding off some kind of perceived danger. But when that danger is mental or emotional rather than physical (such as a tiger about to pounce), your cortisol levels may remain chronically elevated, which means that you remain in a state of heightened awareness and are unable to go back into rest-and-digest mode. Your stomach acid levels might go down, digestive enzyme production will decrease, and your digestion will either speed up or slow down, leading to constipation or diarrhea as well as being bloated and gassy.

But there are other ways in which the relationship between SIBO and your brain is complex. When my first gastroenterologist (Dr. Run-Three-Miles) prescribed an antidepressant for me, I was beyond insulted, thinking he was telling me that my symptoms were all in my head. What I didn't know at the time is that the majority (as much as 95 percent) of the mood-influencing neurotransmitter serotonin is made and stored in the gut. Abnormal levels of serotonin in the gut have been associated not only with mood disorders but also with several gastrointestinal problems, including IBS. Healthy serotonin levels are important for digestive functioning—increased serotonin levels can cause diarrhea, and decreased levels lead to constipation. Knowing this, it makes sense that there is a direct connection on a chemical level between your brain and your gut, so I guess I really should forgive that long-ago gastroenterologist. But the lesson to be learned from my experience is, not only does your doctor need to know what they're talking about, but they also need to be a good communicator.

If he or she isn't communicating as well or as clearly as you would like, you need to ask more questions. In fact, you should never be afraid or embarrassed to question anything you don't understand.

In terms of the gut-brain connection, it is equally important to know that the walls of your digestive system are also home to your "second brain," the enteric nervous system (ENS), whose main role, as Dr. Jay Pasricha explains it, is "controlling digestion, from swallowing to the release of enzymes that break down food to the control of blood flow that helps with nutrient absorption to elimination." Dr. Pasricha is the director of the Johns Hopkins Center for Neurogastroenterology, whose research on the enteric nervous system has garnered international attention. "The enteric nervous system doesn't seem capable of thought as we know it, but it communicates back and forth with our big brain—with profound results," he adds.

Until quite recently it was assumed that your gastrointestinal problems were caused by your emotional issues—you know, like "Snap out of it. You're going to give yourself an ulcer." But now we know that it is a two-way street: your mental state can affect your gut, but your gut can also affect your mental state. And yet, despite what we've discovered about the gut-brain connection, many people are still being told that whatever is bothering them is all in their head. Are you depressed? Feeling depressed about feeling depressed? Your gastrointestinal problems could be the reason.

### The Vagus Nerve and Stress

One of the most important connections between your brain and the enteric nervous system in your gut is the vagus nerve. If your vagus nerve isn't functioning properly, it could be contributing significantly to both your emotional and your gastrointestinal problems. It is the tenth cranial nerve that runs from your face through your chest and down to your abdomen, sending signals all along the way. It acts like a kind of information superhighway between your brain and your gut.

In the previous chapter we talked about your migrating motor complex and the role it plays in sweeping all the leftover debris out of your small intestine when you've finished digesting your food. The MMC functions when you're in rest-and-digest mode. Being chronically stressed actually inhibits the migrating motor complex. And if you're a stress eater or someone who turns to food for comfort, you might be constantly snacking, which doesn't give your migrating motor complex the break it needs to sweep leftover food particles out of your small intestine.

But even being temporarily stressed, such as when you're about to make a speech or take part in a competition, can slow down or disrupt the digestive process, leading to either diarrhea or constipation until the stressful situation has passed.

In fact, stress, in and of itself, is not as simple as it might seem. Pleasurable situations can be as stressful as unpleasant ones. Getting married is an obvious example, but going on vacation might be another. Sometimes eating unfamiliar foods while you are in a new place can give you diarrhea, or you can experience vacation constipation. Being away from home can be stressful even if you're having fun. I experienced this myself when I was on my honeymoon and spent ten days in Hawaii with my husband. The long flight, the change in time zone, and just the excitement of getting married were enough to wreak havoc with my digestion.

Stress can also manifest physically, as a tensing of your muscles. Have you ever been told you're walking around with your shoulders next to your ears? That's stress! And, finally, stress is a two-way street. If you have ongoing gastrointestinal problems, the persistent discomfort can add to your stress and anxiety.

The vagus nerve is key for putting your body into rest-and-digest mode, so if it isn't working properly, the result will be that you'll remain in fight or flight; you'll be feeling more stressed and anxious; you won't be digesting properly; your stomach won't empty; and your MMC won't kick in, so the bacteria in your small intestine will have more food to eat and ferment, causing you more SIBO symptoms.

In addition, if your vagus nerve isn't working the way it should, possibly because you're under too much stress, you could develop leaky gut, which means that toxins are able to escape through the intestinal wall and enter your bloodstream.

So how do you know whether your vagus nerve is doing what it should?

A doctor can test its function by using a cotton swab to "tickle" the back of your throat, which ought to make you gag. If your gag reflex isn't working, there's a good chance that your vagus nerve isn't doing its job. But there are some simple things you can do to stimulate it.

Because the vagus nerve is connected to your vocal cords and the muscles at the back of your throat, singing, humming, chanting, and gargling can activate these muscles and stimulate it, according to Dr. Datis Kharrazian. Something fun to try is to sing really loudly in the shower. Some people also gargle before swallowing when they drink water. There are also several handheld devices you can hold up to your neck to stimulate the vagus nerve, and I, personally, have found acupuncture to be incredibly helpful for getting into a parasympathetic state.

## SIBO AND BRAIN FOG

Brain fog is a symptom of SIBO that I have experienced personally and found incredibly disturbing. I'll never forget the day when, for a short period of time, I actually seemed to lose the ability to form words. I remember the expression on my husband's face as he saw what was happening. We were both just plain scared. I was unable to utter a cohesive sentence and literally slurred my words. There have been many days when I felt as if my head were swimming and I wasn't able to hang on to a thought or stay focused on what I was doing. Occasional brain fog while appearing on TV was a nightmare.

Your experience of brain fog may be different from mine. Perhaps you struggle to recall words, or you forget your to-do list, or maybe you get in the car, zone out, and forget where you're going. Some people forget how to spell a word or do simple math. People forget names, book or movie titles, or don't remember what day it is or what they were about to say. Any one of these things can happen to any one of us every now and then, but with SIBO it can be more pervasive and persistent—and therefore more disturbing.

If you have trouble remembering things or concentrating, even slurring your words from time to time, you probably wouldn't immediately connect those problems with the issues going on in your gut. I certainly didn't. But then I learned that too many endotoxins—the outer layer of bacteria—could be responsible for some of these feelings of fogginess. Gram-negative bacteria, the most common type in the world, can be found in your gut, and their cell walls contain lipopolysaccharide (LPS), which is an endotoxin and one of the most potent inflammatory substances known to man. When you have an overgrowth of bacteria in your small intestine (SIBO), and those bacteria die (either through treatment or on their own), they release their LPS. Your body absorbs it, and that triggers an inflammatory response that can be damaging to your kidneys, your liver, and your cardiovascular system. It can cause any number of conditions, from skin issues and joint pain to gut pain, according to microbiologist Kiran Krishnan.

And if the LPS makes its way into the brain, it has been shown to cause cognitive impairment in mice and a range of behaviors, including anxiety, drowsiness, and general depression, many of which are considered to be similar to the symptoms of neurodegenerative disease in humans.

The trigger for brain fog might also be histamines, which are created or increased by the overgrowth of bacteria in your small intestine—that is, SIBO.

## The SIBO-Histamine Connection

Histamines are chemicals your immune system creates in response to allergens in your body. If you're allergic to pollen, for example, you'll probably get a stuffy, runny nose. If you have a mosquito bite, your skin will swell, turn red, and itch. Those are histamine reactions causing inflammation. To counteract them, you might take an antihistamine such as Benadryl.

You can also have a histamine reaction to certain foods, which may indicate there's something going on in your gut, and SIBO may be the culprit. If you have a rash or severe brain fog, you could have a histamine intolerance related to your SIBO. If you get your SIBO under control, chances are you will also gain control of your histamine problem.

## THE EFFECTS OF PROBIOTICS—BOOM OR BUST?

Probiotics are live bacteria that are intended to support and/or increase your health and well-being. They are also one of the most controversial topics in the SIBO community. They're polarizing—not just philosophically but also in terms of practical experience. Some people are able to resolve all of their symptoms with probiotics alone. In fact, I know many people who have had total SIBO remission from introducing the "right" probiotic.

Others, however, are totally miserable on probiotics and confused as to why they seem to be so helpful for someone else. And because every person's gut microbiome is unique, there's no guarantee that what worked for some other person will work for you.

Many studies have shown that probiotics can help boost your mood as well as your cognitive function while lowering levels of stress and anxiety. However, at least one somewhat controversial study done by Dr. Satish Rao and his colleagues at the Digestive Health Center at the Medical College of Georgia at Augusta University, which was published in the journal *Clinical and Translational Gastroenterology,* has linked not only brain fog but also extreme bloating to taking probiotics. Previous research had already found that too much D-lactic acid in the bloodstream can temporarily interfere with cognitive functions, which creates brain fogginess. And, according to Dr. Rao, "probiotic bacteria have the unique capacity to break down sugar and produce D-lactic acid. So if you inadvertently colonize your small bowel with probiotic bacteria, then you have set the stage for potentially developing lactic acidosis and brain fogginess." The problem, according to Dr. Rao, is that probiotics increase the number of bacteria in your gut and, therefore, increase the amount of D-lactic acid you produce.

Naturopath, nutritionist, and probiotic expert Dr. Jason Hawrelak believes there are several mechanisms of action that could explain how probiotics can benefit SIBO patients. Some probiotic strains are known to have "selective antibacterial action," which means they could potentially help kill some pathogenic bacteria. Some strains are also known to help stimulate the migrating motor complex. Others help reduce visceral hypersensitivity, which can cause the pain SIBO patients feel in their gut. And, finally, some probiotics can enhance secretory IgA, the major antibody found in bodily secretion that helps control bacteria populations in the gut.

Bottom line, if probiotic bacteria affect the bacteria you already have in your body, they could, ultimately, help control everything from your weight to your mental health. Clearly, more research needs to be done, but I believe this is an area of investigation that holds promise for SIBO sufferers.

For now, I think the most important takeaway about probiotics is simply that there is not a one-size-fits-all answer. Some people with

SIBO find them extremely beneficial while they just make others feel worse. If you want to try probiotics, you'll have to be prepared to go through some trial and error. But that can be painful on more than one level, because good-quality probiotics can be quite expensive! To hopefully save you some hassle, I have put together a list of probiotics that are often cited as good for those with SIBO, as well as some of my "best practices" for choosing a probiotic.

## Your Probiotics Buying Guide

What to consider when buying probiotics:

**Check the strength.** Look for those that contain at least one billion CFUs (colony-forming units) per strain. If you choose a probiotic that has multiple strains, be sure there are at least one billion CFUs of each. Research has shown that the effective dose of each probiotic is unique, but experts like Dr. Jason Hawrelak consider one billion CFUs to be a good starting point unless specific research has demonstrated that a particular strain is effective at a lower dose.

**Look for an expiration date (and don't use expired probiotics).** The live bacteria in probiotics will die off over time—for that reason, manufacturers can only guarantee a certain amount of CFUs for a certain length of time. All probiotics expire, so don't buy one without an expiration date.

**Follow storage guidelines.** Not all probiotics require refrigeration, but those that do need to be kept cool because getting too hot can kill all the beneficial bacteria. I was intrigued to find that many of the doctors I spoke with didn't care about keeping them refrigerated. My advice is to follow the label for temperature guidelines, and if one is so sensitive that it can't be at room temperature for very long, it's probably not going to live long enough in your body to make it all the way to your intestines. This is one important reason why I prefer to buy most probiotics at my health food store rather than online. If you're ordering probiotics online, you might want to choose one that is shelf-stable, such as a spore-based probiotic.

**Look for strains.** The best probiotics will list specific strains, not just species, on the label. This usually looks like a collection of letters and numbers after the species name. Not all probiotics include this information, but it's useful to have because probiotic benefits are strain specific.

**Take it at the right time.** There's a lot of controversy about the right time to take probiotics, but naturopathic physician Dr. Mona Morstein recommends taking them with meals for optimal results.

The following probiotics have been well studied and shown to be useful for people with IBS and/or SIBO.

- Megaspore: a spore-based probiotic containing very hardy strains that can survive the stomach acid and arrive intact in the small intestine. Visit sibosos.com/microbiome-labs to learn more.
- *Saccharomyces boulardii*: a yeast-based probiotic that is ideal for people with SIBO, IBS, immune deficiency, travelers' diarrhea, and more.
- Jarrow Formulas Ideal Bowel Support 229v: ideal for people with IBS, abdominal pain, and bloating.
- Visbiome: for people with IBS symptoms, IBD, and other more severe intestinal dysbiosis.

- Metagenics UltraFlora Acute Care: for people with functional GI symptoms who tend toward constipation and have slow intestinal transit.
- NOW Foods Clinical GI Probiotic: for people with functional GI symptoms who tend toward constipation and have slow intestinal transit.
- Align: for IBS patients and other functional gut disorders.
- BioGaia Protectis: for people with methane-type SIBO.
- Doctor's Best Digestive Health 2 Billion: has been shown to help with diarrhea-type symptoms.
- Culturelle Pro-Well Health & Wellness: a well-studied option for people with IBS and other digestive symptoms; the Health & Wellness formula within the Culturelle line does not contain any prebiotics. Prebiotics feed the good bacteria in your gut, but they are problematic for people with SIBO because they are also food for the overgrown bacteria in your small intestine, which ferments them, creating gas and thus aggravating SIBO symptoms.

The active strain of probiotic in Health & Wellness is *Lactobacillus rhamnosus GG*, and you can find it in most major drugstores. In 2017 several studies showing its efficacy were published, and *L. rhamnosus GG* is now considered the most researched probiotic in the world.

## DEALING WITH GRIEF

SIBO can be overwhelming emotionally and impact many aspects of your life. It is perfectly normal to grieve the loss of your health and your routines. Here are some feelings you may be experiencing:

- Body performance grief. The body you'd always counted on is now letting you down.
- Lack-of-diagnosis grief. You feel terrible, but no one knows what's wrong with you.
- Diagnosis grief. You have a diagnosis and it sounds really bad.
- Food grief. You are missing all the foods you love that you can't eat and think you can never eat again.
- Lifestyle grief. You know you have to change the habits that bring you comfort, but you miss the way you used to live.
- Lack-of-spontaneity grief. You now have to be regimented and pay attention to so much all at the same time.

There may be other issues and changes in your life for which you are also mourning. Don't be afraid of your grief; don't discount it. It really is real.

## Look for Online Support

Many people turn to online SIBO support groups to help work through their grief and gain information. I have a SIBO group on Facebook with more than fifteen thousand members that has been immensely helpful to so many people. If you find that connecting with other people who have SIBO is helpful to your healing, join us at https://www.facebook.com/groups/SIBOSOSVirtualSummit/.

As with almost everything related to SIBO and underlying conditions, there is something of a "chicken or the egg" issue here. At least one relatively recent study published in the *Indian Journal of Psychological Medicine* found that because anxiety and/or depression are so often associated with IBS (which means, in effect, with SIBO), gastroenter-ologists should be screening patients for these problems so that they can treat them and improve both outcomes and patients' quality of life.

## How You Can Cope

For all of us living with SIBO, having a mindset for healing is an im-portant part of the process. But maintaining that positivity isn't always easy. The mental and emotional effects of SIBO can be overwhelming. I know, because I've experienced them. When I first determined to begin my journey to wellness, I became laser-focused on my health. At the time, I felt bad enough that I was almost forced to do this just to be able to get through the day. I told myself that it was a privilege for me to be alive and on this planet, and that, to be worthy of that privilege, I had to make this commitment to take good care of myself and put myself first. At least that's how I felt on the good days, and even then, it wasn't always easy for me (and isn't easy for most people, in my esti-mation). It's a commitment I've had to reaffirm from time to time when I temporarily lost my way and had to get back on the healing path.

### Try Not to Panic

I know. That may be a lot like telling you not to think of pink elephants. You have all these symptoms and you don't know why. You begin to think maybe you have cancer. Then your doctor tells you it's not a big deal, just something you'll have to learn to live with. Really? You keep thinking you're coming close to finding an answer, but the answer never seems to materialize. You find something that helps a little, but it isn't the complete answer. The things other people say work for them don't help you. You sometimes wonder if it really is all in your head. At times you feel isolated, lonely, and misunderstood, to the point where you go into full-blown panic mode. The panic, of course, just makes your symptoms worse, so you panic even more. And so on and so on . . .

If you've never felt that way, I'm truly happy for you. If you know exactly what I'm talking about, my heart goes out to you, because I've been there myself.

Sometimes I'm still overwhelmed with anxiety, and when that happens, I generally react either by ramping up the number of treatments I'm trying or by slamming on the brakes and not doing anything because nothing seems to be working and I don't know what to try next. Sometimes the guesswork involved is as difficult to deal with as the symptoms.

Very often just naming what's happening is enough to stop me from spiraling into panic. And having someone you can talk to, even just to say "I'm feeling panicked and hopeless right now," can also help immensely. The best way I've found to keep myself sane is to try to stay in the moment and check in with myself throughout the day: "Okay, how's my mindset? Have I remembered to eat when I was supposed to? Have I taken some time for yoga or meditation?" Having a kind of checklist of things I can do to support myself really helps me stay organized and keeps me on track. Even having a hobby or interest that has nothing to do with my SIBO gives me something to focus on when focusing on my gut health starts turning to panic.

It isn't always easy, but taking it one step, one treatment at a time, instead of worrying what might happen ten steps from now, generally keeps me from throwing myself over the woe-is-me cliff. And it also helps me know what's working and what isn't.

It's tempting to want to try everything at once, or to get frustrated when something doesn't seem to be working the way you think it should and moving on to another supplement or another treatment. The problem with that is, when something goes wrong or triggers a symptom, you're going to have a hard time figuring out what it was. As gut health expert Dr. Michael Ruscio once told me, "It's tempting to try to do it all at once and get there quickly. But if you can slow down a little bit, run these mini-experiments, and listen to your body, then you can learn." Slow and steady will win the race.

But again, if you're feeling panicked all the time and nothing seems to help, you really need to see a professional. Just because SIBO and IBS symptoms aren't all in your head doesn't mean that a good therapist or psychiatrist can't help you work through the very real life mental and emotional problems they can cause.

## Unexpected Advice: Declutter to De-stress

One of the most unexpected and valuable pieces of advice I ever got was to clean up, throw out, organize, and fix what was broken. Literally get your house in order. As herbalist Summer Bock once explained to me, consciously you may not even notice anymore that the board on which you hang your keys has been crooked for months because it needs a new screw, but subconsciously you do. "Every time you walk by an unfinished project it is traumatizing your brain."

I've found this to be particularly true when it comes to items related to my health journey. At one point I had a massive stash of half-used supplements and probiotics that I had tried in good faith, but they just didn't work for me at the time. But what I didn't consciously realize was that every time I looked at them I was reminded of failed treatments and money spent on things that didn't help me. I felt discouraged and resentful. It made me feel that even though I was trying so hard, nothing was working for me.

The silliest part was that I knew I would never use the remaining capsules. Some of them were even expired! But as bad as I felt about keeping them, the thought of throwing them all away felt even worse. The day I finally worked up the courage to trash them was incredibly freeing.

The same rule applies to anything you bought to improve your health that didn't work out. Kitchen appliances, food, books, anything. You don't have to be wasteful: Give it away, donate, sell, or recycle whatever you can. Letting those things go creates space—mentally, physically, and spiritually—for new ideas and answers to come in.

And while it is vitally important to put yourself first, one thing I've found to be an essential part of doing that is to maintain as normal a life as possible, to take the time to be with supportive friends and loved ones, and, in general, to maintain a balance between self-involvement and involvement with society. In the beginning, I found that I became a kind of monk with virtually no social life at all. But, with time, I came to understand that part of the healing process is finding a way to be in the world (not isolated from it) as a person with SIBO. So much of our social life revolves around food that finding a way to be with friends could be challenging. How about going for a walk? There are a lot of things you can do that don't involve worrying about your digestion.

To view the references cited in this chapter, please visit healingsibo.com/references.

# CHAPTER 3

# Your SIBO Medicine Cabinet:
# Simple Remedies for Symptom Relief

In this chapter, I'll cover many of the over-the-counter herbs, supplements, and medications you can find in drugstores or health food stores or online, and other strategies you can use at home when you are experiencing a flare-up or just not feeling great. Keep in mind that you may need to experiment with these suggestions to find the ones that work best for you, or the right combination. They are not meant to be cures or, in most cases, for long-term use.

Dr. Siebecker has divided these remedies into categories according to symptom, but you'll find that some of them show up in more than one place. That's because one symptom—bloating, for example—may be caused by gas, which then creates another symptom, such as pain from muscle cramps.

## BLOATING

Bloating is a symptom that can be ever-present for sufferers of SIBO. But there are ways to find real relief.

## Activated Charcoal

Activated charcoal absorbs gas and is also used for poisoning because it absorbs toxins. You can buy it in most health food stores and take two pills every two to three hours, but don't take them with food or at the same time as any medications. So that raises the question: How long should you wait after eating? Like many SIBO patients, I digest food slowly, so I try to wait at least two hours (which is what's generally recommended) to be certain that I'm taking the charcoal on an empty stomach.

If you're curious about how long it takes for food to move through your system and be eliminated (which is different from how long it takes you to digest what you eat), look for the black stool that you may be producing from taking the charcoal and count backward. Or try eating sesame seeds or poppy seeds. Even people with a perfectly healthy digestive system will find whole seeds in their stool. A study done by the Mayo Clinic found that for healthy adults it takes about forty-eight hours (give or take) for foods we eat to be fully eliminated.

The other issue here is that charcoal may cause constipation. One way to deal with that if it happens is to take magnesium oxide at night before bed to counteract the constipation. (See more about magnesium under "Constipation" on page 50.) I'd suggest starting with the dosage recommended on the bottle and increasing it as necessary until you get the desired results. Don't worry about taking too much; the worst thing that could happen would be that you get diarrhea, but based on what I've heard from other SIBO patients, most people are too cautious with magnesium and, therefore, don't take enough.

I've taken the charcoal and experienced miraculous results. One dose can do the trick.

## Atrantil

Atrantil is a type of antioxidant called polyphenols developed by gastroenterologist Dr. Ken Brown that has been clinically tested and proven to help relieve constipation and reduce bloating caused by methane. Visit sibosos.com/atrantil to learn more.

## Gas-X

You can take Gas-X as needed. It breaks up the surface tension of the gas bubbles and turns large bubbles into smaller ones that may pass more easily.

## Iberogast

Iberogast is like an old folk remedy your grandmother might have told you to take. It is a formulation of nine medicinal herbs in liquid form that originated in Germany. Dr. Siebecker calls it the German version of Pepto-Bismol. It smells like licorice and has an herbal flavor some people love and others hate. Personally, I hate the flavor, but I find that it provides a lot of relief. It works as a prokinetic, stimulating motility of the small intestine to help get rid of the gas that may be trapped there.

Dr. Siebecker recommends Iberogast again and again because it helps alleviate not only gas but also many of the other symptoms of SIBO, including pain, nausea, bloating, constipation, and diarrhea. You can take it before you eat, while you're eating, after eating, or at bedtime. According to Dr. Siebecker, if something's bothering your gut, take it (even if you hate the taste, as I do). You can take the drops directly on your tongue, or you can mix it with water or orange juice, which is what I do. Some people like to mix it in just a little bit of liquid and down it like a shot of whiskey, but I prefer to dilute it in a larger amount of juice to mask the flavor even more.

The first time I used Iberogast was when Dr. Siebecker and I were filming our SIBO patient course, the SIBO Recovery Roadmap. I was feeling unwell that day after traveling, and the Iberogast worked in minutes to make me feel better. I've been a believer ever since.

You probably won't find Iberogast at your local drugstore, but it's sold in many vitamin and herb stores, and you can also find it online. I usually buy mine from Amazon. Many people swear by Iberogast and in my experience it does help. For dosing, follow the directions on the label. One caveat: Iberogast is not recommended if you're using opioids.

## PAIN

Pain may not be the first symptom you think of, but for many people it is the reality of living with SIBO. The pain is almost always caused by muscle cramps or muscles contracting against the gas. Or it can also be caused by visceral hypersensitivity.

### Is Visceral Hypersensitivity Increasing Your Pain?

In medical terms, visceral hypersensitivity (VH) means "decreased thresholds of stimuli perception generated from the gastrointestinal tract." In common English it is an increased sensation in your organs—in this case specifically the organs of digestion. Someone with SIBO or IBS detects pain at a lower level and responds to it more intensely than other people. And there is substantial evidence to show that this is a problem commonly associated with IBS and SIBO.

In addition to feelings of pain, this also applies to feelings of being bloated. People with VH may feel full and bloated when there is no obvious distention of their stomach. Or they might feel a general tenderness or soreness in their entire abdomen. I've heard some people say that because of their VH, they can't wear any sort of tight or restrictive pants.

So, what causes that? Once again, it's complicated. It could be inflammation in the gastrointestinal tract, whether due to bacterial imbalances, dysbiosis, or SIBO; permeability of the gastrointestinal tract; particular infections; or hormonal imbalances. It could also be related to the mind-gut connection in a way we don't completely understand just yet. As a result, treatments are also complex and can include anything from pre- and probiotics to mind-body medicine, acupuncture, even abdominal massage, and, of course, treating the SIBO.

In the end whatever calms down that hypervigilant nervous system allows people to experience less pain and less visceral hypersensitivity. So, there's another very important reason for exploring other problems that may be complicating your SIBO.

## Kava Kava and Black Cohosh

Kava kava and black cohosh are both herbs that work as muscle relaxants. They come in both capsule and tincture forms. Tinctures generally are faster-acting because any time you take a liquid it is absorbed quicker than a pill or a capsule.

Often used to relieve stress and anxiety and to promote sleep, kava kava is well known to alleviate twitching muscles. Black cohosh is often used to alleviate the symptoms of menopause. But they both can also do wonders for SIBO pain caused by muscle cramps or contractions.

## Peppermint Oil or Peppermint Tea

Peppermint is a smooth-muscle relaxant and has antibacterial qualities. Whether you drink it in tea form or take an oil capsule will depend on where your pain is. According to Dr. Siebecker, if the pain is high up, such as underneath your ribs, try drinking strong peppermint tea or take it in tincture form. If the pain is lower down in your abdomen, at or below your belly button, take enteric-coated peppermint oil (ECPO) in capsule form. Actually, I often like to take capsules alongside a glass of peppermint tea to bring relief to my whole abdomen.

Dr. Siebecker recommends IBgard, a peppermint oil capsule formulated for IBS that has little beadlets inside the capsule and is supposed to act even lower down than the regular capsules. It has some good studies behind it, and the claim to fame is that it won't make you burp.

One of the problems with peppermint oil is that it can relax the lower esophageal sphincter between the stomach and the esophagus, which can worsen acid reflux. So it's definitely not recommended for people with acid reflux, but even people without reflux can have a problem with it. IBgard, because it releases farther down, often doesn't do that.

## CONSTIPATION

Constipation is another signature symptom of SIBO, and one of the most uncomfortable.

### Osmotic Laxatives

Osmotic laxatives draw water into the large intestine, which makes the stool softer and creates the urge to move your bowels. These are different from stimulant laxatives and are generally considered less habit-forming. In general, they are magnesium-based. In the last section, I mentioned taking magnesium to counteract the constipating effects of activated charcoal and how it works.

There are several different types of magnesium. Glycinate, citrate, oxide, and L-threonate are just some of the types you might find on the store shelf. So which one is best for constipation? A lot of people like magnesium citrate, but Dr. Siebecker recommends magnesium oxide because it is not absorbed as well by your body, which means that it works better as a laxative. If you're looking for the other benefits of magnesium—such as helping to alleviate anxiety, lower blood pressure, relieve migraine headaches, and improve cardiovascular health—you might consider taking another more absorbable type as well as magnesium oxide for constipation.

If your constipation is severe and chronic, Dr. Siebecker's recommendation is to start with 1,000 mg of magnesium oxide, and you may need to increase that to 1,200 mg or even 1,500 mg. Again, as with most things related to SIBO, it depends on the individual. And you need to take it three nights in a row to give it a chance to do the job. It's best to start with a lower dose and work your way up until you're having regular bowel movements. If you get diarrhea you've taken too much and need to lower your dose. But I've found that most people err on the side of taking too little and then think it didn't work.

Miralax is also an osmotic laxative that is available in many drugstores. I prefer magnesium, but some people swear by Miralax. The medical community seems to really love Miralax, and many doctors rely on it for colonoscopy prep.

## Hemorrhoids and Constipation

Hemorrhoids are at the top of the list of things people don't want to talk about. But if you're constipated, they can be a real problem, and there are solutions.

According to Dr. Crane Holmes, a naturopathic gastroenterologist and primary care physician in Portland, Oregon, one of the primary causes of hemorrhoids is straining during bowel movements, so one of the primary forms of both prevention and cure is to make elimination easier. He describes a hemorrhoid in terms of a balloon. The first time you blow it up, it's fairly stiff and difficult to inflate, but the more pressure you apply, the easier it gets.

He prescribes magnesium to help resolve constipation and, therefore, eliminate straining. Basically, he says, the kind of magnesium that works best for his patients is very individualized, so he doesn't recommend any specific type. What he does recommend, however, is that you take it in one dose at bedtime rather than splitting the dose between morning and evening, because he believes doing that is more likely to produce an easier bowel movement in the morning.

Other methods used to reduce the hemorrhoids and alleviate pain range from topical treatments such as herbals or the old standby Preparation H to old-fashioned sitz baths to more invasive interventions right up to surgical removal of the hemorrhoid.

The main point, however, is that preventing or alleviating constipation is the best and surest way to prevent or alleviate hemorrhoids.

## Insoluble Fiber

I'm sure you've heard that fiber is a good way to combat constipation, and, in fact, it does work for some people, so it's worth a try. Compared to other types of fiber, insoluble fiber is good because it's not very fermentable and is, therefore, less likely to be turned into gas, which could then cause more bloating and other problems. For some people with SIBO, however, it can actually make symptoms worse and aggravate more than it helps. If you find that's the case for you, just stop taking it. The only way to know is to give it a try.

Nut butters, nut flours, peas, and green beans are good sources of dietary insoluble fiber, or you can get it in the form of a powder such as Cellulose from NutriCology. But if you don't respond well to foods like nuts, you probably won't feel well taking an insoluble fiber supplement.

If you do take a supplement, I really recommend starting with a small amount and slowly increasing the dose over time. If you discover that you don't respond well to it, you'll be much happier having taken a smaller dose rather than a large one that leaves you feeling gassy and bloated for several days!

## Iberogast

As we've already discussed, Iberogast is very helpful for motility in both the large and small intestine. It's not a laxative, but if you're using it for other symptoms, you may find it helps constipation, too.

## Probiotics

Probiotics are known to help regulate bowel movements, but they can be tricky for SIBO patients because they very often make bloating worse, and because, as we've already discussed, a lot of people with SIBO are also histamine intolerant. Since many probiotics can trigger a histamine response, they might aggravate somebody with histamine intolerance. That doesn't mean probiotics are bad, or even bad for people with SIBO; it just means you need to be thoughtful about which one you choose.

First of all, if you do take a supplement form of probiotic, you should, as I've said, get one that doesn't also contain prebiotics.

Prebiotics are often mixed with probiotics to help the probiotics do their job. If you're not sure, these terms on the label indicate that your probiotic contains prebiotics:

- FOS (fructo-oligosaccharide)
- GOS (galacto-oligosaccharide)
- Inulin
- Dextrin
- Lactulose

In addition, you need to be sure your probiotics do not contain d-lactate acid, because people with SIBO often have d-lactate acidosis, which means that too much of this type of acid is already being absorbed into the bloodstream, and you don't want to make the problem even worse. Look for probiotics that are labeled as being d-lactate acid free, such as the one made by Custom Probiotics. See "Your Probiotics Buying Guide" on page 36.

Note that a new study done on the probiotic called *Lactobacillus reuteri,* found in the probiotic BioGaia Protectis, has shown that it lowers methane and helps with bowel movements, and so could help with constipation. BioGaia Protectis is marketed as a probiotic for infants, but adults can use it, too. It's sold as a liquid and you just dispense the drops on your tongue. I order it from Amazon.

Also see "Your Probiotics Buying Guide" on page 36.

## Learn How to Poop

When people are constipated, they often strain to have a bowel movement, which, if done incorrectly, can be really dangerous and lead to hemorrhoids and fissures. So yes, there is a wrong way and a right way to poop. Most people take a deep breath, push while holding their breath, and then exhale. (Imagine you're pushing right now and you'll see what I mean!) But, as Dr. Steven Sandberg-Lewis explains, when you're pushing to get something out, you need to breathe before you can contract your abdominal muscles. (You can think of this as pushing out a baby, if that helps you to understand the concept.) First take a deep breath, then breathe out as you press down. Here's the key: If you run out of air, stop bearing down and take another breath. You'll find that doing this doesn't allow you to create as much pressure, but that's exactly the point. You don't want to build up so much pressure that you develop hemorrhoids or a hernia. You want to do things effectively but safely.

## Water

This might seem obvious, but some people don't realize just how dehydrated they really are. Staying hydrated throughout the day is one of the best ways to ease constipation, but you really need to pay attention to how much you're drinking for it to be effective.

There are many apps you can get on your phone to help you keep track of your water intake throughout the day. I like Waterlogged, Daily Water, and WaterMinder. You can also move rubber bands from your wrist to your water bottle every time you finish a full quart-size bottle. Having four rubber bands on the bottle at the end of the day signifying four quarts consumed is a great feeling both emotionally and physically.

Drinking water is great, but you don't want to be drinking out of plastic water bottles all day. Buy a reusable water bottle instead. There are several available on Amazon that have a cultlike following because they are leak-proof, easy to clean, and attractive. I mention easy to clean because you really need to keep on top of sanitizing the cap and opening of these bottles. They are breeding grounds for bacteria and germs when used daily without a serious cleaning. When I travel, I ask the hotel to run my water bottle through their dishwasher, or I use my own electric coil to boil water and pour it in and around the bottle daily.

### Potassium

Potassium can help bring water into the large intestine and loosen the stool a little bit. It's gentler than some of the other constipation remedies, but some people respond really well.

Fresh homemade cucumber, carrot, or tomato juice, bananas, or avocado, if you can tolerate it, are all good food sources of potassium.

Other remedies for getting things moving include stool softeners such as docusate sodium and docusate calcium, coffee enemas, and glycerin suppositories, the last of which are especially handy to use when you're traveling.

## DIARRHEA

It may seem counterintuitive, but many of the same things that help with constipation will generally also work for diarrhea, because, in effect, they are both working to regulate bowel movements.

### Insoluble Fiber

Follow instructions under "Constipation" on page 52.

### Activated Charcoal

See under "Bloating," above, and remember that this can cause constipation, thus counteracting diarrhea.

### Over-the-Counter Medications
#### Imodium

#### Pepto-Bismol

Taking Pepto-Bismol might make both your tongue and your stool
turn black temporarily. That's because of the bismuth in the Pepto-
Bismol. It's perfectly normal and it will pass.

### Food Remedies

Cut down on fats, fruits, and vegetables, all of which can increase
diarrhea.

## NAUSEA

Poor digestion causes all kinds of unpleasant symptoms including feeling sick to your stomach much of the time.

### Iberogast

Iberogast can help if you're nauseated because it helps the downward
movement of the gastrointestinal tract and lack of motility.

### Ginger

Ginger is famous for being an antinausea herb and often used for morning sickness in pregnancy.

Ginger comes in many forms, any of which would be helpful. In
fact, many people have told me that putting a two-inch chunk of

peeled fresh ginger in a glass of hot water with lemon and sipping it all day helps control nausea.

## Acupressure

There is an acupressure point on your inner arm near your wrist (called point pc-6, which you can find online to locate exactly) that you can press with your fingers to relieve nausea.

# ACID REFLUX

Sometimes called heartburn, acid reflux, which causes a burning sensation in the upper abdomen, is often associated with SIBO.

## Baking Soda

Dissolve ½ teaspoon of baking soda in 4 ounces of water and drink. It works by neutralizing the acid in your stomach and provides immediate relief.

## Tums

What can I say? They work for occasional use, but if you're chewing up several a day, as I was for a while, it's a sure sign you have some additional problem that ought to be addressed.

## Iberogast

Iberogast is also great for acid reflux!

## Herbal Bitters, Hydrochloric Acid Pills, or Apple Cider Vinegar

Low stomach acid (which may be the result of having taken antacids over a long period of time) can prevent you from breaking down and absorbing some nutrients. But the reason some people have acid reflux is because they have too little stomach acid. It's counterintuitive, but we need enough acid to strengthen the lower esophageal sphincter

(LES). The LES acts like a kind of trapdoor between the end of the esophagus and the top of the stomach. When the stomach is empty it opens to let food in; when the stomach is full, it closes. But when we have too little stomach acid, the sphincter just hangs open, allowing what's in the stomach to back up into the esophagus.

There are three different remedies you can take that help stimulate acid: herbal bitters, hydrochloric acid pills, and apple cider vinegar.

The actual taste of the herbal bitters on the tongue helps stimulate the production of stomach acid, which, in turn, strengthens the esophageal sphincter and, therefore, reduces acid reflux. In some cultures, people eat certain seeds at the end of a meal to promote proper digestion. You can buy the bitters in most liquor and health food stores.

Hydrochloric acid (HCl) pills and apple cider vinegar work in the same way.

One caveat, however, is that you should start with a very low dose, because otherwise you might start to produce *too much* stomach acid before the sphincter has gotten a chance to close. If even that low dose causes you pain, you might actually be producing too much (rather than too little) stomach acid and should be taking an antacid such as Tums or baking soda instead. As I keep saying, all of this is really a matter of trial and error, and figuring out what works for you.

One other important note: According to Dr. Pimentel, in high doses, HCl may act as a hydrogen donor, which can then, potentially be converted into methane gas. If you have high levels of methane, you'll want to be aware of this when trying HCl, as there is the potential that HCl could make you feel worse. Most people find HCl helps them, and it is definitely worth exploring.

### Alginate

I particularly like an unusual treatment for acid reflux involving alginate, which is a kind of seaweed raft—and no, I'm not making that up. It's a substance made from brown algae and calcium carbonate that mix with stomach acid and form a gel. The gel sits on top of the food you've eaten and prevents reflux. You can buy it as a supplement in capsule form and take it in place of antacid. It's more common in the UK than in the United States.

## GENERAL INDIGESTION

SIBO is, after all is said and done, a digestive problem whose symptoms can flare up at any time in many different ways. Therefore, it's a good idea to have an arsenal of products on hand that are known to alleviate all sorts of indigestion.

### Digestive Enzymes

Very often, when people have digestive issues, it's really not the food that's the problem. It's the person's inability to break down the food. Most of the time, giving the body the right tools allows real healing to take place. Digestive enzymes help you break down your food into smaller particles so that they're easier to digest. Your body makes digestive enzymes, but, like stomach acid, they can be depleted as a result of stress, a poor diet, or illness. In those cases, taking supplementary enzymes can help. They are best taken before your meal. Brands to look for include ProZymes, Vital-Zymes, Holozyme Digest Platinum, and Digest Gold.

### Chewing Gum

Chewing gum can help relieve digestion upset, especially ginger gum. Dr. Sam Rahbar, cofounder and medical director of Los Angeles Integrative Gastroenterology and Nutrition, advises chewing gum after meals to help stimulate the vagus nerve and improve digestion. Just be careful of what gum you choose, since many artificial sweeteners can provoke SIBO symptoms. I like the brand Simply Gum, which is sweetened with a small amount of cane sugar. Some people also can tolerate gum sweetened with xylitol, since it is used in such a small amount.

## Hydrochloric Acid (HCl), Herbal Bitters, or Apple Cider Vinegar

See under "Acid Reflux" above.

## Colostrum

The first milk produced by the mammary glands of mammals after the birth of a child, colostrum contains immune-enhancing properties, and recent studies have shown that taking supplements of bovine colostrum, which is similar to human colostrum, can be beneficial to gut health and particularly for decreasing leaky gut. I've taken it and found it to be very soothing and very healing, as have many others. Look for a brand that is lactose-free.

## Probiotics

See under "Constipation and Diarrhea" above.

# OTHER NATURAL TREATMENTS

Other treatments I've found to be helpful include castor oil packs, acupuncture, acupressure, and reflexology, all of which you can use to alleviate pain, constipation, diarrhea, nausea, bloating, and acid reflux, as well as to help with detoxification and relaxing your vagus nerve.

## Castor Oil

Castor oil comes from the castor bean, which is native to India. Castor oil packs are an ancient treatment still used all the time by naturopathic and Ayurvedic physicians, and they are extremely helpful for reducing inflammation and increasing motility. You put about 2 tablespoons of organic castor oil on a soft cloth and place it on your abdomen (I wrap plastic around my middle to hold the pack in place. You need to keep it there for a least an hour or even overnight. The only problem is that the oil is thick and sticky, and it can get a bit messy, so you shouldn't be trying this when you're wearing your favorite nightclothes. But don't let that deter you. The first few times you will probably think it isn't working. Give it a few days. It's a marvelous detoxifier and helps with the bloat!

Castor oil can also be taken orally, generally 1 to 3 tablespoons. Taken that way, it's a very strong laxative. The packs take a little longer to work, but they're gentler, and so I prefer that method. I also love the oil for removing makeup and as a beauty treatment for my cuticles and skin.

## Acupuncture

Acupuncture uses very fine needles inserted at specific points on the skin that are believed to be related to particular organs and areas inside the body. It has been used in traditional Chinese medicine for more than three thousand years and helps maintain healthy digestion by modulating the expansion and contraction of muscles in the GI tract. It can help improve motility and activate the parasympathetic nervous system so that the vagus nerve functions more efficiently. It has absolutely helped improve my own overall health and well-being. Each time I leave an acupuncture session, I feel hopeful and as if I'd just gotten eight hours of sleep.

## Acupressure

Acupressure is based on the same principles as acupuncture but applies pressure to acupuncture points rather than using needles. At least one study done in China has shown that it can improve gastrointestinal motility in women after an abdominal hysterectomy.

## Reflexology

Reflexology is a kind of acupressure applied to specific points on the feet. It is known to help treat both constipation and diarrhea in people with irritable bowel syndrome (a.k.a. SIBO).

What I love about all three of these remedies is that they provide virtually instant relaxation and reduction of anxiety. You can do both acupressure and reflexology on yourself, wherever and whenever you want or need the relief.

Hypnotherapy is another way to alleviate both psychological and physiological symptoms of IBS, whether or not it is caused by SIBO. It won't help you to find or treat the root cause or your SIBO, but it will make you feel better in the here and now.

## TIPS FOR HELPING YOU GET THROUGH THE DAY

Here are some tips that I've found help make my life easier even (or particularly) in difficult times.

- Take your medicine at the same time every day.
- But of course, if there's a reason why you can't take them at the same time every day, it's still better to take them when you can than it would be to not take them at all.
- Use timer caps and other reminders. I buy timer caps from Amazon for my medications that let me know the last time I opened the bottle, and I also set timers on my phone. Both are particularly helpful if you're having brain fog or if you're just so busy that you just forget. Just remember to keep them someplace where you're going to hear them!
- Keep everything together. Keep all your meds and supplements together in one place so you don't have to go searching when you need them and you don't forget something because it isn't right there in front of you.
- Keep a travel stash, too. I also keep mini supplies of all my pills by my bed and in my purse just in case I've forgotten to take my evening meds or I'm rushing out the door and don't have time to take them before I leave home. It's just a good idea to give yourself as many chances as you possibly can to stay on track.
- Try to eat your meals at the same time every day. Doing this will stabilize your metabolism and make sure that you're leaving

enough time between meals for your migrating motor complex, which should be resweeping every ninety minutes when you're fasting between meals, to do its job. Eating even a little bit stops the process, which is, incidentally, why snacking between meals is not advised if you have SIBO. Even getting ready to eat— smelling your food, looking at it, and thinking about how great it will be to eat—gets the saliva flowing, which means digestion is starting, and that, too, can turn off your MMC. Dr. Mark Pimentel suggests waiting four to five hours between meals, just in case your small intestine motility isn't what it should be. I find that eating (and taking supplements) at 8 A.M., 2 P.M., and 8 P.M. is the best schedule for me. You'll have to figure out what schedule is going to work best for you; just remember to leave time for that all-important mini-fast between meals. Since consuming any calories at all turns off the MMC, that means no cream in your coffee. Some people drink black coffee or tea or some other sugar-free, zero-calorie drink that won't interrupt your MMC.

- Go outside. Get out in the sun for a little while each day, but remember to always use sunscreen!
- Meditate—twice a day if possible. There are apps and techniques to help you get started. Headspace (www.headspace.com) has award-winning audio meditations, and Self-Realization Fellowship (www.yogananda-srf.org) is my personal favorite source of mediations. I highly recommend both of them.
  - Meditation is part of my daily practice—and the key word here is practice, because it's not going to be perfect, maybe not ever. That's just life. But, after years of meditating, and comparing my life before meditating to my life after, I truly believe that meditation is the key to a better life.
- Try to get some mild exercise every day. I'm not saying you have to run three miles, but I'm sure you already know that moving your body is good for you. It helps regulate your lymphatic system and improves digestion.

- Make time to be with friends. If you book the date in advance, it will give you something to look forward to.
- Make your bathroom a safe haven. You want the rest of your home to be attractive, so don't forget the bathroom. Make it a place you enjoy being. It should be a comfortable temperature. You might want soft music playing, and it should smell good. The point is to create a tranquil, comfortable, and private space. Is your toilet at a comfortable height? If not, you might look into getting a new toilet installed (this is not as expensive as it may sound) or installing an elevated toilet seat or a frame over your existing toilet that elevates your feet off the ground. Are you worried that people can hear what you're doing in there? Even a fan or noise machine could help with that.
  - There are many small changes you can make to reduce bathroom stress, which will put your nervous system into a parasympathetic state, thus also improving your digestion. Traditional chemical-based air fresheners can have a negative impact on highly sensitive people. So, go easy on the artificial scents. There are so many essential oil choices and high-quality diffusers. And Poo-Pourri is a brilliant invention that covers all kinds of odors and can give your bathroom a spa vibe.
- Get enough sleep. Getting good sleep is important because it gives your MMC time to do its job properly. Sleep has been really getting a lot of attention in the media these days, which makes me very happy, because I think preparing for a good night's sleep is one of the most overlooked and easily fixed mistakes or habits you can make. What works for me is to be sure the room is dark enough, wear an eye mask if necessary, use good sheets, and experiment with pillows until you find one you really LOVE. Sleep.org also suggests that you keep your room temperature at between 60 and 67 degrees Fahrenheit, because your body temperature drops slightly to initiate sleep and keeping your room in this range helps facilitate that. Also, take the time to become

aware of the noise level in your room. There are now actually apps that allow you to check the decibel level in your environment. When I did that, I was absolutely shocked by the traffic noise I've never consciously noticed before. I started wearing earplugs, and after a day or two of getting used to them, I slept more soundly than I had in ages.

- If you've been told that you snore, you might want to be tested for sleep apnea, which not only could be affecting your sleep but could actually be putting your life at risk.

- And, finally, you could also take melatonin supplements, which not only promote better sleep but also have been shown to, at least potentially, alleviate symptoms of IBS (and, therefore, presumably SIBO). Melatonin is available in many forms, including tablets, liquids, and even gummies. I personally like Physica Energetics Melatonin Liposome Spray because, by spraying it on your tongue, it is absorbed directly into the bloodstream, bypassing the stomach—which means it works more quickly, it doesn't require drinking water, and the dosage is easy to adjust.

To view the references cited in this chapter, please visit healingsibo.com/references.

# CHAPTER 4

# Change Your Diet to Change Your Life

Changing your diet is the fastest way to start feeling relief from your SIBO symptoms. Diet alone can't cure SIBO. I repeat: diet alone can't cure SIBO. This is one of the most confusing aspects of this condition. The only exception is the Elemental Diet, which is a treatment more than a way of eating (more on that to come). While some people can manage their symptoms successfully through diet, in order to actually eradicate the bacteria for good, you also need to use one of the treatment options I'll be discussing in Chapter 6. Still, diet is enormously important. If you change how you eat today, you will feel better today.

In addition to being extremely effective, changing your diet is empowering, because you can do it at home and it gives you a sense that you have some control over your own health. How, what, when, and where you eat is an integral part of your lifestyle. So, in addition to being life-sustaining, food is social and highly emotional, which is why it can be hard to make changes. It's important to be patient with yourself as you work to make shifts mentally, physically, and logistically.

## CARBS ARE FERMENTABLE FOODS

The general rule is that to relieve your symptoms you will need to limit your intake of carbohydrates, which are fermentable foods. That is because SIBO bacteria feed on carbs and ferment them into gas, which not only causes bloating but also triggers many of the other gastrointestinal problems you've been living with for so long.

Most of us think of carbohydrates as those sugary and starchy foods—cookies, cakes, ice cream, pasta, and potatoes, to name a few. But there's also sugar (lactose) in milk products and in fruits (fructose). In fact, all vegetables, starchy or not, are carbohydrates, and there are also some carbs in meat products. What this means is that carbs are really hard to avoid entirely, and, in fact, you'll see that ripe fruits, non-starchy vegetables, and nuts are allowed on the plan I outline in Chapter 5. And honey is also allowed because it contains simple sugars that are absorbed quickly before bacteria can ferment them (clover honey appears to be the type that most people tolerate best).

Carbs, in and of themselves, are not "bad." In fact, the diet I recommend does not cut out carbs completely. Instead, it shows you how to limit your intake of fermentable carbs to a quantity you can tolerate without exacerbating your symptoms. If you feel worse after a meal—any meal—it is probably because the meal contained more fermentable carbohydrates than you could tolerate.

## You Don't Need to Eat the "Perfect" Diet

The good news is that, because changing your diet is really about alleviating symptoms, not curing the disease, you don't have to worry about the fact that if from time to time you eat something that isn't on the diet, you'll be making your condition worse. In other words, you don't have to be perfect to get results. That said, however, the more compliant you are, the better you'll feel. And because of that, most people find they really don't want to cheat once they realize how good they can feel just by sticking with it.

In general, you should stick with foods that are low in fermentable carbohydrates and easy to digest, so that they don't feed the bacteria in your small intestine or put an additional burden on your already-compromised digestive system. This means that they should be low in FODMAPs. FODMAP stands for fermentable oligo-, di, mono-saccharides and polyols, which are forms of sugar found in carbohydrates that feed the bacteria in your small intestine, thus causing the SIBO symptoms we know and hate: gas, bloating, and diarrhea or constipation.

In this book I use the terms "low fermentation" and "low FOD-MAP" interchangeably.

It's confusing to think of high FODMAP foods like apples, pears, some legumes, and wheat products as foods you should avoid, since they are healthy for most people. But try to forget everything you know about what is healthy and what is unhealthy and approach this new way of eating with a totally open mind. But, at the same time, do remember that the foods excluded on this diet are not "bad foods." There are simply foods that do or don't work for you right now. For example, avocado may upset your stomach now, but that doesn't make it bad, and, hopefully, you'll be able to reintroduce it at some point.

Every person and every case of SIBO is different, so no two people will follow the diet exactly the same way. There will be some foods you're allowed to eat but choose not to. Since I'm a vegetarian, all the recipes in this book are vegetarian, but you can add one of the proteins listed on page 217 if you so choose. Some people have strong reactions to particular foods that others tolerate well, and vice versa, so even with the excellent guidelines provided in this book, experimentation with your diet will be key. And, as you get better, you will want to try reintroducing more foods. The more diverse foods you are eventually able to eat, the more diverse your gut microbiome, which is important for overall health.

## FOODS THAT HELP REDUCE SIBO SYMPTOMS

Again, everyone is different, but most people seem to do well eating the right amounts of the foods listed below. If you're in doubt or need more help, please reach out to a nutritionist who is knowledgeable about SIBO. Working with a nutritionist who really knows this condition could be one of the most valuable things you do during this journey. I have found that many, if not most, patients don't make this investment, but when I finally did, I wondered why I hadn't done it sooner. Working with my nutritionist, Kristy Regan, was a game changer for me. I not only felt better, but I also was much more satisfied with the food I did eat. I tried things I hadn't thought I would like, and I did! One of the big treats was pitaya (dragon fruit). If you like sweet treats, dragon fruit is delicious and even better than ice cream, when frozen and served with fresh fruit.

A nutritionist can help you be certain you're eating as diverse a diet as possible. Remaining on a very restricted diet for too long can damage the diversity of bacteria in your microbiome and, therefore, leave you vulnerable to other problems. The more diverse your diet, the more likely it is that you will be able to stick with it because you won't be bored. Here are the kinds of meals and foods that are the foundation of a healing, diverse diet:

Pureed soup, such as the Delicata Squash Soup (page 158), or Shivan's Soothing Soup (page 160).

Food that is well cooked, soft, and preferably pureed (think baby food), such as the Pureed Carrots (page 186). The point is that you want your food prep to do as much of the breaking down as possible to start the digestion process for you. We'll be talking more about what those specific foods should be in Chapter 8.

24-Hour Yogurt (page 138), because this process removes the lactose, which is fermentable.

Fruits that are not highly fermentable, such as bananas, canta-loupe, grapes, kiwi, oranges, pineapple, and strawberries, but not highly fermentable fruits (even though they may be otherwise healthy, such as apples, cherries, dried fruit, peaches, nectarines, plums, mango, pears, or watermelon). If you have trouble digest-ing fruit, try cooking it, because the cooking starts the digestion process for you. I love to caramelize bananas in maple syrup or clover honey with a dusting of cinnamon, which also satisfies my sweet tooth.

Smoothie bowls, such as the Acai Smoothie Bowl (page 140).

Clover honey (as well as alfalfa, wildflower, and raspberry) because of the ratio of fructose to glucose molecules. According to Dr. Siebecker, the ratio of fructose to glucose in these forms of honey is 50:50, so they are potentially less reactive for people with fructose intolerance than other types of honeys that have a higher fructose content. SIBO can cause fructose intolerance, but many people with SIBO also have an underlying fructose intolerance, so, one way or another, it's wise to choose foods with less fructose.

Interestingly, the inability to absorb fructose in the intestinal tract has been associated with symptoms including bloating, flatulence, and loose stools, which are the same symptoms SIBO can cause.

Chocolate—hooray! Just be sure that it's dark chocolate, which is relatively low FODMAP and doesn't contain any lactose. You can eat about 30 grams, which is just over an ounce, or about a third of a standard-size chocolate bar.

## FOODS THAT CAN TRIGGER SIBO SYMPTOMS

Remember: There is no actual evidence to show that what you eat actually increases the number of bacteria in your small intestine. SIBO is not caused by eating fermentable carbohydrates (even in large quantities). So don't worry that you're making your SIBO worse—or that you gave it to yourself—by eating the wrong foods. All that eating the wrong foods can and does do is to make your symptoms worse. You'll know rather quickly if you've eaten something you shouldn't have.

Remember that when you have SIBO your body is basically a small brewery, so, to put it simply, you want to stay away from foods that are highly fermentable because they feed the overgrown bacteria in your gut and are hard to digest. As I've already mentioned, some—in fact many—of these foods are actually very healthy for most people. Whole grains, beans, and most fruits and veggies are just some of the foods that are great for healthy microbiomes but tough on those with SIBO.

So, what should you avoid to help keep SIBO symptoms under control?

Raw foods in general. Cutting out raw salads is probably the easiest thing we can do to reduce our symptoms right away. Raw vegetables contain a lot of fiber that is difficult to digest; cooking them begins to break down that fiber for you. So, stay away from the crudités and cook your vegetables very well (which is probably exactly the opposite of what you've been taught). And Dr. Siebecker suggests that you also cook the vegetables you put in your green smoothies, assuming you make smoothies.

Whole grains because they have lots of fermentable carbs and require more work to digest. Again, exactly the opposite of what healthy-eating advocates generally suggest. In fact, many people with SIBO find that white bread is the only kind of bread they can tolerate.

## Autoimmune Disease—the Link between Gluten and SIBO

I can't really talk about whole grains without talking about gluten. Gluten is the collective name for a group of proteins found in a variety of cereal grains but primarily in wheat.

In people with celiac disease, gluten causes an autoimmune reaction that damages the lining of the small intestine. Celiac disease (both undiagnosed and diagnosed) often coexists with SIBO.

You can be sensitive to gluten without actually having celiac disease. The medical term for this condition is non-celiac gluten sensitivity (NCGS). NCGS does not, in and of itself, create long-term damage to the small intestine, but it does cause an autoimmune inflammatory response that can create all kinds of problems not only in your gut but in other parts of your body as well.

High-fiber foods, which are generally plant-based, including fruits, vegetables, and grains. The reason is that most fiber is fermentable and feeds the bacteria you're trying to starve. Fiber is indigestible to humans but not to bacteria. So, under normal circumstances, the undigested fiber goes down into the large intestine, where the bacteria will digest it, ferment it, and make good things out of it that help keep us healthy. They also make a little bit of gas in the process, which we excrete, usually without even noticing. That's normal. What's not normal is that, with SIBO, the bacteria are in the small intestine, where they don't belong. So even though the bacteria are doing what they're supposed to do, they're now harming rather than helping us.

But I don't want to tell you to *not eat* fruits and vegetables. What you need to do is cook them well to break down the fiber before you eat them. I eat lots and lots of fruits and veggies every day. I simply make sure that I stick to those that are lower FODMAP, cook them (I rarely eat raw veggies), and watch my portion sizes.

## A Tip for Bean Lovers

Many types of beans are off-limits if you have SIBO, but a bean-lover foodie friend gave me this tip for making them less fermentable.

Add a strip of kombu, which is a kind of seaweed you can buy at any Asian grocery or in health food stores, to the water when you cook your beans. It helps break down the raffinose, a kind of sugar in beans that bacteria love to ferment, so it also reduces the amount of gas the beans will produce. Just remember to throw out the kombu with the cooking water. Don't eat it.

In addition, soaking dried beans overnight or for up to 24 hours can make them much more digestible. Beano or Beanzyme (the vegetarian version) can also help reduce symptoms when you eat beans.

Fermentable fruits and vegetables, including garlic and onions, because they contain high levels of FODMAPs, which are fermentable in the intestine and can, therefore, cause bacteria to increase.

Apples, even though you've undoubtedly heard all your life that an apple a day keeps the doctor away. Apples are not only high in fiber, they are also highly fermentable because they contain fructose—a double whammy for people with SIBO.

Dairy products, including milk and milk products, soft cheeses, and most yogurt (except for 24-Hour Yogurt [page 138]), because they contain lactose, which is a type of sugar (that is, a carbohydrate) that is highly fermentable.

You could try lactose-free dairy products or even taking a lactase pill to help you digest the lactose. In addition, many cheeses do not contain any lactose. Read the label; if the sugar content is 0, there isn't any lactose, which is the form of sugar found in dairy products. But aged cheeses, even if they don't contain lactose, may contain histamines, which is an entirely different issue that could also exacerbate symptoms. And, of course, if you're vegan, you can just ignore this whole section because it doesn't affect you.

Alcohol, even in moderate amounts, has been associated with increased incidence of SIBO. A glass of champagne at a celebration is different from a glass of red wine every night to unwind. In general, alcohol isn't good for you. It's hard on your liver; it's a depressant, slowing down parts of your brain that are responsible for cognition and response time; and there is a clear relationship between alcoholism and clinical depression. In many instances, it appears that the depression led to the alcohol abuse, but drinking a lot can also harm your brain and lead to depression. In the end, this is a highly personal decision driven by many factors aside from how it impacts your health.

Finally, as I've already said, quantity counts. Just because you've made a giant batch of something you really like that isn't supposed to exacerbate your symptoms doesn't mean too much of a good thing can't be bad. For example, I like carrots, and eating one or two of them is fine for me. But a big cooked carrot salad would cause symptoms for most people with SIBO even though carrots are not very fermentable.

In the end, the goal is to eat as many different foods as you can in portions you can tolerate. Determining what those are, and what your limits are, will require trial and error. Here comes the pep talk: you're going to need curiosity, a sense of adventure, endurance, creativity, and determination. It's the understanding that this is a journey of discovery and you are an explorer in a land that may, at least at first, seem foreign, and perhaps even hostile to you. Just keep exploring and keep an open mind; what seems odd and unworkable to you now will likely become more familiar and friendly going forward.

## ADDITIONAL FOOD TIPS

Portions matter. Sometimes a little of something—one-eighth of an avocado, for example—-is okay, but too much will push you over the edge because it's too fermentable. Many people think that if they can tolerate something, and they like it, they have carte blanche to eat it to their heart's content. But that simply isn't true.

Don't worry about what other people are eating. Some people who have SIBO can eat an egg with no negative effects, some people can tolerate coconut while others can't, and the same is true of other foods.

Combinations matter. Eating one fermentable food at a meal could be fine, but eating it in combination with another fermentable food could be one fermentable too many. As just about any SIBO sufferer or clinician will tell you, sometimes you really need to try it to figure out what works for you.

Keep your ingredients simple. Stay away from foods that contain garlic (although garlic-infused oil may be okay for you), are super-spicy or acidic, or that have too many components. Not only will that make it harder for you to digest, but if you have a negative reaction it will also make it more difficult to figure out which food is causing it.

Space your meals four to five hours apart. You want to give your stomach time to empty and your migrating motor complex a chance to sweep out whatever is left in your small intestine after digestion before you send more down the tube.

If you're on the go, take your own food with you. That way you'll always have something SIBO-friendly to eat. There are many reusable lunch boxes and bags you can put in the freezer so that your food will stay fresh for most of the day after you take it out. Two brands to look for are PackIt and Yeti. At the risk of repeating myself, I want to remind you that it's important to keep your food fresh in order to avoid food poisoning.

Strategize when you're eating out in a restaurant. When you are eating out, there are a few different factors to consider. If it's a celebration, such as a birthday dinner, you may decide it's worth it to have your slice of cake and a latte and pay the price the next day. But if you've been feeling really good for a while and don't want your symptoms to flare up, you have a few options. Eat before you go, and if your companion(s) comment that you're not eating, you can say you had a late lunch or that your doctor has told you that you need to be on a really restricted diet. That will usually shut people up. The phrase "doctor's orders" has saved me on many occasions.

Of course, if you're with good friends who are aware of your situation, no explanation may be necessary. But if it's a business lunch or a meal with people you don't know well, what has worked for me is to arrive early and speak with the server or host. Explain that you're on a very restrictive diet and would like to order in advance so that you don't become the focus of the conversation at the table. Most restaurants will be happy to work with you, so long as you explain the problem politely.

Be sure that you're hydrated. Drink at least eight cups of good filtered or bottled water a day. Water helps to move things through your system and get them out of your gut. Some people are actually constipated simply because they're dehydrated. And if you have diarrhea, you may also be dehydrated because of all the water you've been losing in your stool.

Luckily, eating a small amount of anything is not likely to have a significant impact on how you feel. That's a very important thing to remember. And experimenting is not going to make your SIBO worse; it may make you *feel* worse for a little while. But if by experimenting you find out that something you thought you couldn't eat is actually great, you'll be expanding your dietary repertoire—and that is a great gut feeling. Plus—the more diverse your diet is, the better it is for maintaining the variety of good bacteria in your large intestine, where you need them to help you maintain optimum health.

To view the references cited in this chapter, please visit healingsibo.com/references.

# CHAPTER 5

# The 21-Day Plan

Now that we've covered the basics of what foods help alleviate symptoms and what foods you should avoid, let's dive into the 21-Day plan. The nutrition plan I outline in this chapter is based on the SIBO Specific Food Guide (SSFG) (also called the SIBO Diet or SIBO Specific Diet). This food guide was developed by Dr. Siebecker and is based on her clinical experience treating SIBO. It combines the recommendations of the Specific Carbohydrate Diet and the low FODMAP diet and is low fermentable. I love this eating guide because it delivers great results, but it's also flexible. You can actually stick to it and live your life.

## OTHER NUTRITIONAL APPROACHES TO SIBO

The SIBO Specific Food Guide has worked best for me, but there are other nutrition plans for SIBO that you may have heard of or that you are experimenting with. Some are more restrictive than others, but all of these diets work for the same reason: They reduce the amount of fermentable carbohydrates you're eating, which, in turn, gives the overgrown bacteria in your gut less to eat! If you are following a different type of eating plan, you can still use the recipes in Chapter 8—just consult the label I've included with each recipe to see whether it is compatible with your particular plan. Here is an overview of the other recommended diets:

The low FODMAP diet was created at Monash University in Melbourne, Australia, to help people with IBD and IBS, and has since been adopted by many practitioners for treating SIBO. The diet includes a restrictive list of high FODMAP (fermentable) foods paired with low FODMAP alternatives. The goal is not to completely eliminate FODMAPs (which would probably be nearly impossible) but to reduce them to a level that allows you to manage your symptoms. After an initial all-low FODMAP restriction period, experimentation of moderate and high FODMAP foods follows to find what is individually tolerated. Staying on the low FODMAP–only diet over the long term can actually disrupt the number and diversity of good bacteria in your microbiome, which is why it's important to not get stuck in the initial restrictive phase.

The Cedars-Sinai Low Fermentation Diet (CSD) was designed by gastroenterologists at Cedars-Sinai Hospital, as the name would suggest. The diet is low fiber and emphasizes the importance of fasting between meals so that the MMC can function properly. Foods like white rice, white bread, and cookies are generally allowed, and vegetables are less restricted than on the low FODMAP diet. Lactose-free dairy (such as lactose-free milk and hard cheeses) are also allowed. If you're feeling overwhelmed by making substantial changes to your eating habits, this diet is a great way to start because it is easy to follow (even when eating out) and is very helpful for many people.

The Specific Carbohydrate Diet (SCD) is one of the oldest therapeutic diets, so some of the foods, such as dry curd cottage cheese, may sound strange or be difficult to find. It is a grain-free, low-sugar, low-lactose diet originally created for the management of celiac disease that is now often used for the treatment of IBS and SIBO. Because it focuses on foods that are easy to digest but doesn't consider FODMAPs, it's generally recommended for people with more moderate cases of

SIBO who can tolerate a wider variety of vegetables than those who are more reactive or have more complicated cases.

The GAPS (gut and psychology syndrome) diet was initially designed for autistic patients as part of a whole treatment plan. It is a variation of the SCD and works very well for people with mood or brain disorders who also have GI disorders, which is not uncommon. But because it is not a SIBO diet, you might need to modify it a bit to eliminate high fermentable FODMAP foods such as avocado and onion. Like the SCD, however, it limits carbohydrate intake and focuses on foods that are easy to digest, so it is likely to be helpful for people with SIBO. It emphasizes animal products, so it is hard to follow if you are vegetarian.

The SIBO Bi-Phasic Diet is Dr. Siebecker's SIBO Specific Food Guide, broken into two phases by Dr. Nirala Jacobi, with some variations. The first phase is intended to reduce symptoms, and the second phase is done in conjunction with SIBO treatment (herbal antibiotics).

## Eating Disorders and SIBO

We can't talk about following any diet for SIBO without bringing up eating disorders. This isn't just an issue for those who have suffered from disordered eating in the past. In fact, the restriction of a SIBO diet, necessary though it may be, can actually lead to the development of an eating disorder.

According to Dr. Siebecker, "When you're on a diet that's so restricted both in scope and in portion size, it could trigger an eating disorder, which is why we try to treat the SIBO and then expand the diet as soon as possible. The goal is to expand the diet as much as we can as soon as we can. More diversity leads to a healthier microbiome, more nutrients, more minerals, and, ultimately, better health overall. In addition, since food is one of our major sources of pleasure, the more foods you can eat without feeling sick, the happier you will be."

Sometimes you need to treat yourself and have a small amount of something you love. If you don't allow yourself to do that, you might just give up on the diet altogether because you can't bear the idea of never tasting that food ever again for the rest of your life. Remember, food doesn't cause SIBO, and occasionally eating foods that trigger your symptoms won't make your SIBO worse, so it's okay to "let loose" sometimes (as long as you're prepared for the short-term flare-up of symptoms that may follow). I find it helpful to plan my treats in advance, because it gives me something to look forward to and also helps to put an "end time" on the treat so it doesn't turn into an entire weekend of eating all the foods that make me feel bad.

With that in mind, the SIBO Specific Food Guide is forgiving, and, unlike many other diets, it's easy for vegetarians to follow.

## Legal and Illegal Foods

The Specific Carbohydrate Diet uses the terms "legal" and "illegal" to differentiate foods you can eat from those you shouldn't. While that sounds pretty straightforward, it is too simplistic.

For instance, many foods are "moderate FODMAP," which means they contain some fermentable carbohydrates. In large quantities, these foods can cause symptoms (as can even low FODMAP foods when eaten in large quantities). But, on the other hand, high FODMAP foods can often be tolerated in small amounts. All of which means that no food should be considered totally illegal, and that kind of black-and-white thinking can make following a SIBO diet more difficult and limiting than it needs to be.

That's why I much prefer Dr. Siebecker's color-coding system, which progresses from green to red, with green foods being the least fermentable and red food the most.

I know I can tolerate most green foods, small quantities of most yellow and orange foods, and even some red foods. No foods are totally off-limits, which, for me, is extremely reassuring.

In the Appendix (page 211) you will find a version of Dr. Siebecker's SIBO Specific Food Guide. To suit my particular vegetarian needs, I simply moved eggs up into the dairy category and listed other proteins at the end, which you can add if you are not a vegetarian. Besides being vegetarian (and delicious), my recipes include starches like white rice, which isn't listed in SSFG, and potato, which is in the red category. However, other SIBO diets include starchy foods—many SIBO patients tolerate them, including me—and they are important for vegetarians.

Dr. Siebecker's instructions include:

- Start with low (green) and moderate (yellow) fermentable foods.
- When you start the diet, and for at least the first week, cook, peel, deseed, and puree all vegetables and fruits.
- Limit moderate (yellow) fermentable foods to one per meal and separate your meals by at least four to five hours.
- The quantities listed are for adult-size portions. When no quantity is given, it means either that the food can be consumed in unlimited quantities or that no specific amount was recommended in the low FODMAP diet at the time the food guide was created in 2014. Note that larger quantities of a particular food may be considered moderate or highly fermentable even when a smaller quantity is low fermentable.

- Tailor the diet to your personal preferences and tolerance level. Trust your body's reactions to particular foods. Just because it is listed in the food guide as red doesn't mean the food will be a problem for you.
- Tolerance levels change over time, so retry foods to which you've previously had a negative reaction.
- Wait until you are feeling better to introduce celery root, rutabagas, cruciferous vegetables, beans, seeds, nuts (including nut flours, butters, and milks), coffee, alcohol, raw vegetables, salads, and some raw fruit.
- Remember that the SSFG is a starting point you can use to help you figure out what to try, not a do-or-die list of foods you must avoid forever.

## THE PLAN

The key to your success is going to be preparation. For those who are used to simply grabbing something on the fly, this will be a huge lifestyle change. It won't be easy, so keep your eye on the prize or the light at the end of the tunnel, to quote a couple of clichés. It's going to require both a mindset and a logistical change because you're going to have to be sure that you always have on hand the food you need/want to eat.

### Before You Begin

Take an inventory of your kitchen. Do you have a good supply of green and yellow foods on hand? If not, stock up! If you've got a lot of red or orange foods, you don't need to panic. You might want to donate or give away anything perishable, but you'll probably be able to reintroduce some or most of these foods in the future, so there's no reason to get rid of foods that will keep for a while on your pantry shelf. Look online for companies that are making low FODMAP foods. And see the Recipe Grocery List (page 122) so that you can shop for the ingredients you'll need for the meal plans.

Some of your old favorites may no longer work for you, but if you get creative, you can find substitutions that will make you feel just as satisfied! In fact, you may even discover some new favorites. Just because you're eating fewer foods doesn't mean you need to eat less. You may just need to be more diligent about getting enough calories—especially protein—each day.

Make sure you have a good supply of SIBO-friendly staples—including garlic-free seasonings, condiments, and salad dressings as well as fresh or frozen fruit for smoothies and your favorite sweeteners such as clover honey or stevia.

One thing you should not be doing is going hungry. Have you ever been hangry—so hungry that you're angry? I have, and I didn't even realize until after I'd eaten something that I'd really just been hungry.

### Apps to Help You Use What You Have

If, like me, you've ever stood in front of your refrigerator or pantry trying to decide what to do with the ingredients you have on hand, using an app that figures it out for you can be just what you need. Simply input the foods you have available and receive a recipe or selection of recipes that use those ingredients. A few options include

- Fridgetotable.com
- Chopchopfamily.org
- Myfridgefood.com

Also, make sure you have all the proper cooking utensils. See the Kitchen Tools List (page 125).

## To Keep You on Track

Here are some strategies for the weeks ahead to keep you going.

- Keep a food diary. I know, it's annoying, but it does work. It helps you learn which foods trigger your symptom and which ones don't. For example, I found that I could eat about 4 tablespoons of avocado, which meant that I actually had to measure the amount. I couldn't just think, okay, you can eat half an avocado, because they come in different sizes.
  - Rebecca Coomes, a SIBO survivor and now a SIBO health coach, says that once she started keeping a "food and mood" diary, she was able to listen to her body and appreciate the clues it was giving her rather than blaming it for what was and wasn't working for her. For example, she'd say, "Thanks, body. So much for those symptoms. That bloating was great because now I know I just can't tolerate pumpkin."
  - Write down what you intend to eat and then write down what you actually did eat. If they're not the same, think about why. A friend came over? You were too busy?
  - Also write down the quantities of what you ate and how you felt afterward.
- If you hate keeping a food diary, use your phone to take a picture of everything you eat instead. The photos will be conveniently date- and time-stamped (and if you don't eat the whole meal, take a picture of what is left over, too). Then you can flip back through photos and see exactly when and what you ate without having to write anything down. A photo won't give you as much data as tracking with pen and paper everything you eat, but it's a great alternative if typical food diaries simply don't work for you.
- Plan your meals in advance. Several days or a week ahead would be ideal, but if you can't do that, even a day in

advance would be helpful. I know that many people suggest planning meals—and even cooking—for a week at a time, but Dr. Sheila Dean taught me that planning twenty-four hours in advance is more realistic for most of her patients. Just plan as far in advance as is doable for your lifestyle. And, of course, don't panic if plans change. You don't want to be so rigid about your meal planning that you can't enjoy a spontaneous lunch date with a friend. This diet is meant to give you back your life, not take it away from you.

- Keep a supply of your favorite fresh herbs. Herbs can add flavor to your food without triggering your symptoms.
- Make big batches of foods that are freezable. If you freeze single servings, you'll always have something that's nourishing and that you like to defrost when you don't have time to cook. There are many cool ice-cube-type trays now available that are modified just for this purpose.
- Invest in a set of reusable food storage containers in a variety of sizes. They are much safer and more eco-friendly than plastic wrap and bags. I've found that square and rectangular-shaped containers fit into my fridge and freezer far better.
- Look for "green" foods in the SIBO Specific Food Guide. These are the foods that are less likely to trigger your symptoms, but don't be stubborn. If you eat a green food and are instantly bloated and gassy, you probably don't tolerate that food just yet. Remove it from your diet for now and try it again later on.
- Start with purees. At first, when your symptoms are very bad, peel, deseed, cook, and puree all vegetables and fruits except for very soft ones like ripe bananas and avocado. Over time, you'll be able to eat them whole, gently cooked, and eventually even raw again.
- Find a reliable way to track your water intake. Remember to stay hydrated.

- Don't let yourself get too hungry. If you are hungry, you'll have a hard time chewing well and eating slowly, and you may even wind up saying "What the hell" and going off the plan. Low blood sugar is not your friend!

## YOUR WEEK-BY-WEEK PLAN AND EXPECTED RESULTS

You'll see that some recipes have items in italic. That means it's a simple recipe I assume you already know how to make, such as a grilled cheese sandwich.

In addition, you will find that some recipes include foods that are not on the SSFG diet but are, nevertheless, SIBO-friendly, meaning that they don't contain any ingredients that are high in fermentable carbohydrates.

You shouldn't go hungry while you're following this guide. Feel free to increase portion sizes to your tolerance, or add more recipes from those listed in Chapter 8 to round out any of the meals. If tolerated, gluten-free bread drizzled with garlic-infused olive oil is one of my favorite additions to any meal.

### Where's the Beef?

I am a vegetarian, so all of the recipes in this book are vegetarian. If you do eat meat, you can add a serving taken from the list on page 217 to any of the recipes.

My favorite vegetarian and SIBO-friendly proteins include firm tofu (silken tofu is higher in FODMAPs), eggs, nut butters, and beans in small servings. As with any food suggested in this book, only eat these if they work for you. Everyone is unique, and foods that don't bother me might be a problem for you.

## Before You Begin Week I

This is the most restrictive week of your diet as you figure out what works for you and get your symptoms under control. Eliminate as many carbohydrates, as much fiber, and as many triggering foods as you possibly can. Steam and/or sauté all your fruits and veggies, or make soups. Your food needs to be predigested as much as possible.

It's also important to immediately start keeping track of what foods you can and can't tolerate. I made a master list of all the foods I liked and could eat (and a separate list of foods I couldn't tolerate). When I was stumped trying to decide what to eat, I could turn to my "good" list for ideas. And, moving forward, I also used my "bad" list to help reintroduce foods I initially wasn't able to tolerate. It was always exciting to move foods from no to yes. Most people aren't reintroducing foods in Week 1, but it is vital to start this list now and keep it up.

It's possible that during Week 1 you might not be able to tolerate all of the recipes I'm giving you here. You might want or need to keep it even simpler, so that if something doesn't agree with you, you'll have an easier time figuring out what food caused the problem. When a dish has lots of different foods in it, it can be very difficult to determine which one is triggering your symptoms. Once you've established your list of well-tolerated foods, you can get back to being creative in the kitchen!

You might actually notice a huge difference in the very first week as you cut out the foods that have been triggering your symptoms. You will probably notice that you're less bloated—which feels good! But even if you don't notice a difference right away, don't be discouraged. You always notice when you're gassy and you bloat, but you may not immediately notice when you don't bloat. So keeping a food diary should also be a reminder to self-assess each day, think about how you feel and whether you feel better or worse.

A word of caution: Week 1 might not go as smoothly as you'd like. Just keep at it. It will be worth it.

## Your Week I To-Do List

In addition to following the meal plan, help support your healing in Week 1 by following the guidance below.

Stock Up on Symptom-Relief Medication and Supplements

Since Week 1 is all about getting your symptoms under control, you should check back through the lists I've provided in Chapter 3 and stock up on symptomatic relief supplies.

Another thing to consider in Week 1 is adding a multivitamin to make sure all of your nutrition bases are covered.

Take a Breath Test

If you haven't already taken or scheduled a breath test, now is the time to do it. Make an appointment and see if your doctor wants you to complete the test in the office or if you can do it at home. Remember that you'll need about twenty-four hours to complete your prep, so take that into account when you're scheduling the test.

### Remember . . .

There's a really good chance—up to 78 percent—that if you have IBS, it was caused by SIBO. Once you've confirmed that, you can eradicate the bacteria—as I'll be explaining in Chapter 6—and take back your life, waving goodbye in the rearview mirror to IBS.

Keep Track

Keep track of the circumstances in which you felt better or worse after a meal and see if you can link the foods you ate to your mood at the time or to a specific life event. Doing that will help you make better choices moving forward.

Remember to also keep up that list of questions that hopefully you have already started. There will surely be issues that come up as you start your new diet that you'll want your doctor to answer. And when you get those answers, make sure you write them down. Gathering data is an important part of this journey.

Set Your Intention

This week is all about setting the intention to heal your body. Make a commitment to yourself to make the necessary changes, but don't be too hard on yourself if or when you make a mistake (which we all do, especially when we're trying something new), and above all, avoid holding a pity party. You have accomplished the most important part: getting started. Let the excitement and enthusiasm you're feeling carry you through the adversities of the first week.

This is a great time to clean out any meds and supplements that didn't work or have long since expired.

### WEEK I

**Monday**

Breakfast: 24-Hour Yogurt (page 138) with clover honey and low FODMAP fruit and nuts

Lunch: Open-Faced Egg Salad Sandwich (page 163) and Pureed Carrots (page 186)

Dinner: Crispy Accordion Potatoes (page 183), Green Goddess Dressing (page 204), steamed vegetable, and protein of choice

**Tuesday**

Breakfast: Refreshing Basil-Cucumber Water (page 129) and Easy Veggie Scramble (page 136, with one or two vegetables only)

Lunch: White Rice (page 179) with leftover steamed vegetable and protein of choice

Dinner: Roasted Delicata Squash with Five Spice Powder (page 185) and protein of choice

**Wednesday**

Breakfast: 24-Hour Yogurt (page 138) with clover honey and banana

Lunch: Easy Mashed Potatoes (page 184) with Pureed Carrots (page 186) and protein of choice (leftovers from Tuesday)

Dinner: Zesty Zucchini Pizza Bites (page 152), Shivan's Soothing Soup (page 160), and protein of choice

**Thursday**

Breakfast: Orange Cinnamon Rice Pudding (page 194) and scrambled eggs with one vegetable

Lunch: Angel Eggs (page 146) with Quick Pickled Cucumbers and Carrots (page 148)

Dinner: Easy Pesto Rice (page 180) with Tapenade (page 206) and Berry Compote (page 141)

**Friday**

Breakfast: 24-Hour Yogurt (page 138) with clover honey and banana

Lunch: White Rice (page 179) with scrambled eggs and vegetables

Dinner: Angel Eggs (page 146) and Pureed Carrots (page 186)

**Saturday**

Breakfast: Leftover Orange Cinnamon Rice Pudding (page 194) and scrambled eggs with one vegetable

Lunch: Easy Mashed Potatoes (page 184) with Pureed Carrots (page 186) and protein of choice

Dinner: Open-Faced Egg Salad Sandwich (page 163) and Pureed Carrots (page 186)

**Sunday**
Breakfast: 24-Hour Yogurt (page 138) with Berry Compote (page 141) and clover honey

Lunch: Leftover Open-Faced Egg Salad Sandwich (page 163) and Pureed Carrots (page 186)

Dinner: Sautéed vegetables topped with Herb Compound Butter (page 205) and protein of choice

## Before You Begin Week 2

You may start to notice a bigger difference in the second week, but then you may begin to doubt your own perceptions—am I really noticing a difference, or is it all in my head? Trust your gut (literally)!

When you start to feel better you may think you can start eating things you know you shouldn't eat. Don't get too far ahead of yourself, but it's okay to start to reintroduce a few ingredients at this stage on a trial basis.

The key to reintroducing ingredients is to do it one at a time, much as you would do on an allergy elimination diet, and give yourself time before testing another new ingredient so that you can track how your body reacts to each one individually. I have heard of people being able to tell within a few minutes to a few hours how they react to a new food, but if you have very slow motility, a window of up to seventy-two hours can be helpful.

## Your Week 2 To-Do List

As you start to feel the positive effects of changing your diet, take this opportunity to look deeper into ways you can enhance your health.

Revisit Your Supplements

A few questions to ask yourself: Which ones have you been taking? Have you noticed any difference in how you're feeling? If they seem to be working, that's great. Stick with them. But if you don't feel any better, and certainly if you feel worse, go back to my list of suggestions and see if there are any you haven't tried. If so, now is probably a good time to give them a try.

Consider Your Health History

Now that you've made it through the first week, it's an excellent time to start deciphering your underlying cause. Go back as far as your memory will allow and write down any health-related events you can recall. Obviously, anything that stands out, such as a broken bone or a hospitalization, belongs on your list, but don't overlook more seemingly insignificant incidents, such as food poisoning or a fall that left a bump on your head. Also, write down if and when you remember taking any prescription medications such as opioids or antibiotics.

If you suspect postinfectious IBS/SIBO caused by food poisoning, ask your doctor about ordering the ibs-smart blood test. Finding your underlying cause will help determine the best way for you to move forward with your healing, and, in my experience, give you a great sense of peace. You'll no longer be wondering "why me?" or "will it always be this way?" You'll know why and you'll have a plan to change things!

To give you some support and reinforcement, this might also be a good time to consider joining a SIBO group online, like my group at https://www.facebook.com/groups /SIBOSOSVirtualSummit. Knowing that there are others out there going through the same thing can be incredibly helpful.

## WEEK 2

**Monday**

Breakfast: 24-Hour Yogurt (page 138) with Berry Compote
(page 141)

Lunch: *Grilled Cheese Sandwich* (not SSFG) with Tapenade
(page 206)

Dinner: Roasted Artichoke Hearts (page 150), Cheesy Baked
Carrot Fries with Ranch Dressing (page 187), and protein of choice

**Tuesday**

Breakfast: Easy Veggie Scramble (page 136)

Lunch: Open-Faced Egg Salad Sandwich (page 163) and Pureed
Carrots (page 186)

Dinner: Zesty Zucchini Pizza Bites (page 152) with protein of
choice, Shivan's Soothing Soup (page 160), and leftover Berry
Compote (page 141)

**Wednesday**

Breakfast: 24-Hour Yogurt (page 138) with clover honey and banana

Lunch: Leftover Zesty Zucchini Pizza Bites (page 152) with
protein of choice

Dinner: Cheesy Veggie Frittata (page 174)

**Thursday**

Breakfast: Leftover Cheesy Veggie Frittata (page 74)

Lunch: Easy Mashed Potatoes (page 184) with Pureed Carrots
(page 186) and protein of choice

Dinner: Spaghetti Squash Lasagna (page 168)

**Friday**

Breakfast: Pureed Carrots (page 186) with cinnamon and scrambled
eggs

Lunch: Leftover Spaghetti Squash Lasagna (page 168)

Dinner: Mexican Baked Potato (page 170)

**Saturday**

Breakfast: 24-Hour Yogurt (page 138) with Berry Compote (page 141)

Lunch: Leftover Mexican Baked Potato (page 170)

Dinner: Roasted Delicata Squash with Five Spice Powder (page 185), steamed vegetable of choice, and protein of choice

**Sunday**

Breakfast: Hard-boiled egg and Pureed Carrots (page 186) with cinnamon

Lunch: White Rice (page 179), steamed vegetable, and protein of choice

Dinner: Crispy Accordion Potatoes (page 183), steamed vegetable, and protein of choice

## Before You Begin Week 3

You know what to eat, it is starting to become a habit, and you are feeling noticeably better. Everything from your mood to your sleep pattern is stabilizing and changing for the better. By the third week most people really do start to notice a pattern of improvement that is steadily building on itself—less bloating, less pain from the bloating, more regular bowel habits. You still have bacteria in your small intestine; you still have SIBO, but you're have fewer symptoms.

You should have a pretty good routine going, so you can start to plan your meals for the following week based on the recipes you now know work best for you.

## Your Week 3 To-Do List

Below are some other things you can do to support your health during Week 3.

Explore Further Treatment

Hopefully you've taken the breath test and have your
results, so, if you haven't already started treatment, now is the
time to decide which way to go.

Let Yourself Feel Good

This week is all about feeling good again! Hopefully,
you're already seeing big improvements in your health,
and you know it's only going to get better from here
on out.

The only "mental trap" to beware of this week is doing too
much too soon. You might get overexcited and start
reintroducing foods and cause a flare-up of your symptoms.
That's normal. Don't beat yourself up about it; just get back
to doing what works, and you'll be feeling good again in
no time.

Not feeling great yet? Don't be discouraged, as this is still
only the beginning of your journey.

Week 3 is about setting yourself up for long-term health,
happiness, and comfort.

## WEEK 3

**Monday**

Breakfast: Frozen Blueberry Yogurt Bites (page 144)

Lunch: Broccoli Cheddar Soup (page 156)

Dinner: Rainbow Veggie Spring Rolls with Almond
Dipping Sauce (page 165) and clover honey, Honey Macaroons
(page 190)

**Tuesday**

Breakfast: Earl Grey Latte (page 132) and Acai Smoothie Bowl
(page 140)

Lunch: Leftover Broccoli Cheddar Soup (page 156)

Dinner: Shepherd's Pie (page 176)

**Wednesday**

Breakfast: Get Going Green Juice (page 128) and Frozen Blueberry Yogurt Bites (page 144)

Lunch: Leftover Shepherd's Pie (page 176)

Dinner: Leftover Rainbow Veggie Spring Rolls with Almond Dipping Sauce (page 165) and Zesty Lime Pie (page 192)

**Thursday**

Breakfast: Nutty Ginger Banana Smoothie (page 130) with added protein powder of choice

Lunch: Leftover Rainbow Veggie Spring Rolls with Almond Dipping Sauce (page 165)

Dinner: Pineapple Fried Rice (page 181)

**Friday**

Breakfast: Honey Lavender Latte (page 131) and Blueberry-Lemon Muffin (page 134)

Lunch: Leftover Pineapple Fried Rice (page 181)

Dinner: Creamy Spinach Artichoke Dip (page 154) with SIBO-friendly crackers, protein of choice, and Ginger Almond Cookies (page 196)

**Saturday**

Breakfast: 24-Hour Yogurt (page 138) with Grain-Free Granola (page 142) and clover honey

Lunch: Delicata Squash Soup (page 158) with Citrus and Roasted Fennel Salad (page 161)

Dinner: Buddha Bowl (page 2) with Green Goddess Dressing (page 204)

**Sunday**

Breakfast: Earl Grey Latte (page 132) and Acai Smoothie Bowl (page 140)

Lunch: Delicata Squash Soup (page 158) with Citrus and Roasted Fennel Salad (page 161) (leftovers from Saturday)

Dinner: Easy Pesto Rice (page 180) with vegetables and protein of choice, and Chocolate-Covered Bananas (page 198)

## And What about the Weeks That Follow?

You can continue on this diet while also continuing to reintroduce more foods as your gut heals and your microbiome improves.

To view the references cited in this chapter, please visit healingsibo.com/references.

# CHAPTER 6

# How to Destroy the Bacteria

We've already talked about some relatively simple remedies you can use—in addition to changing your diet—for symptom relief. But, while diet and symptomatic relief can help you feel better in the short term, they won't get rid of the overgrown bacteria in your small intestine.

But if you can actually get rid of the bacteria entirely, you will take care of most of those symptoms, including bloating, once and for all. This chapter is dedicated to the treatments that can kill the overgrowth and actually get rid of SIBO.

There are three kinds of treatment you can use to do that: pharmaceutical antibiotics, herbal antibiotics, and the elemental diet.

When you're starting treatment, you need to know that it will probably be a marathon, not a sprint. Most SIBO patients need more than one course of treatment or even one kind of treatment. What works for someone else may not work for you. Having that mindset from the start will help you go the distance.

## PHARMACEUTICAL ANTIBIOTICS

There are three main types of antibiotics used to treat SIBO: rifaximin (brand name Xifaxan), neomycin, and metronidazole (a.k.a. Flagyl).

Many people don't want to take antibiotics. Most of us have heard that we all take too many of them too often, but there are good reasons to try these particular antibiotics for treating SIBO. The treatment for hydrogen is rifaximin alone, while the treatment for methane is rifaximin along with either neomycin or metronidazole.

### New Treatment on the Horizon

In an exciting new development as of this writing, Dr. Mark Pimentel continues to be hopeful that a modified-release form of lovastatin called SYN-010, a medication initially used to lower cholesterol, could inhibit the production of methane and thus help with the constipation type of SIBO.

### Rifaximin

As Dr. Siebecker explains, rifaximin is a very special antibiotic. Rifaximin does not have the same side effects as a typical antibiotic. Unlike other antibiotics, it is not absorbed into the bloodstream. Therefore, it is less likely than typical antibiotics to create side effects such as urinary tract infections, and studies have shown that it does not cause yeast overgrowth. This is important to know, because pharmaceutical antibiotics are famous for indiscriminately destroying everything in our microbiome, particularly in the large intestine where all the good bacteria live. Rifaximin, on the contrary, does not do that, and, in fact, has been shown to *increase* two types of good bacteria, lactobacilli and bifidus, in the large intestine. And, finally, it acts as an anti-inflammatory by shutting down what is known as the nuclear factor kappa B (NF-κB) inflammatory pathway, a protein complex that plays a key role in regulating the immune response to infection.

So, in addition to being nontoxic and safe, rifaximin actually increases good bacteria in the large intestine and reduces inflammation.

A benchmark clinical trial conducted in 2010 found that those people treated with rifaximin alone had a 62 percent success rate in eradicating SIBO.

The icing on the cake is that very few people appear to be allergic to rifaximin, and most do not develop a resistance to it, so that it will continue to work if multiple courses of treatment are necessary—as they often are with SIBO.

## Neomycin and Metronidazole

Neomycin and metronidazole are both typical antibiotics. They can cause unpleasant side effects and impact the microbiome, and yet a lot of gastroenterologists use them for the methane type of SIBO. According to Dr. Siebecker, neomycin is similar to rifaximin in that it, too, stays in the intestines rather than being absorbed into the bloodstream. But, unlike rifaximin, it works on the large intestine as well as the small intestine, and it does decrease beneficial bacteria in a way that typical antibiotics would do. A rare side effect of intravenous neomycin, but not oral pills, is hearing loss. If you already have hearing loss, talk to your doctor about this before starting neomycin.

Generally, a course of antibiotics takes about two weeks, and it can take up to six rounds of treatment to reduce your bacteria load to a negative test result.

The standard dosing of rifaximin for hydrogen-type SIBO is 1,650 mg per day (that is, 550 mg taken three times a day) for fourteen days.

The dosing for methane-type SIBO is 1,650 mg of rifaximin (550 mg taken three times a day) for fourteen days PLUS 1,000 mg of neomycin (500 mg taken two times a day) for fourteen days.

For rifaximin and metronidazole, the dose is 1,650 mg rifaximin (550 mg taken three times daily) for fourteen days PLUS 750 mg metronidazole (250 mg taken three times a day) for fourteen days.

I know antibiotics can be controversial, but when used correctly they are one of the most effective treatments for SIBO.

### Herbal Antibiotics (Antimicrobials)

Herbal antibiotics are another treatment option and have been shown to be as effective as pharmaceuticals, if not more effective. They generally take longer to do the job. They usually take about a month to work instead of the average two-week course of pharmaceutical antibiotics.

Herbal antibiotics are often the first choice for most naturopathic physicians, and, personally, I love the idea of herbs as a treatment—particularly if your symptoms are mild enough for you to tolerate the four-week treatment period and/or you prefer doing things naturally. I often prefer natural remedies, and I tried killing off my bacterial overgrowth with herbs. But while I did feel better, because my case of SIBO is complicated, the herbal antibiotics didn't work for me as quickly or efficiently as I had hoped they would.

Other than the fact that they're natural, two great things about herbs are that they don't require a prescription, and if you don't have insurance, they are generally less expensive than pharmaceutical antibiotics. I should point out, however, that because you can buy them over the counter, you might be tempted to start self-treating without first taking the breath test to confirm that you really have SIBO. Not a good idea! As I've already mentioned and will be discussing in detail in Chapter 7, SIBO can have many underlying causes and/or co-conditions and can also present in the same way as other illnesses, some of which might actually require an entirely different kind of treatment. And for those same reasons, you should retest after you've been taking the herbs for thirty days to be sure your bacterial load is decreasing.

According to Dr. Siebecker, the four herbs most often used to treat SIBO are:

- Neem (a.k.a. Indian lilac), which is a member of the mahogany family
- Herbs that contain berberine (found in goldenseal, Oregon grape, barberry, coptis, and philodendron and available in combination

in supplement form), which activates an enzyme in the body that plays a major role in regulating metabolism
- Oregano or oregano oil
- Stabilized allicin extract, which comes from garlic and is particularly helpful for the methane type of SIBO. (Garlic itself is off-limits on most SIBO diets because it contains FOS—fructooligosaccharides—which are fermentable in the intestine and can, therefore, cause bacterial fermentation, but allicin extract does not.)

These herbs are generally taken in combination, since, individually, they perform different functions.

Dr. Siebecker recommends taking two of these herbs in combination and at the following doses for a period of four weeks per course—with the understanding that more than one course of treatment may be necessary.

- Neem (she recommends Neem Plus from Ayush Herbs because it contains triphala, a traditional Ayurvedic formula that seems to help with small intestinal motility: 6 pills a day, either 2 pills, three times daily or 3 pills twice a day
- Berberine: 5 grams or 5,000 mg per day (this is more than most people take, and winds up being more than 10 pills, so check the milligram listings carefully. Many round down to 9 pills/day or just under 5,000 mg): 3 pills three times a day
- Oregano (she recommends Biotics Research A.D.P., which comes in tablet form and is less irritating to the digestive tract than the oil in capsule form): 2 pills three times a day
- For methane: allicin (she recommends Allimed, also sold as Allimax Pro, as the formula with the highest potency of 450 mg allicin/pill): 6 pills a day, either 2 pills three times a day or 3 pills twice a day. This is used for methane SIBO along with any one of

the other three herbs. Use link https://www.allimax.us/?AffId =40 and code SIBOSOS for a special discount.

As with determining what foods you should or shouldn't eat, deciding on the combination of herbs that will be right for you can take some trial and error. If you're someone who tends to react to almost everything you put in your mouth, maybe start with a low dose. If you have a bad reaction, stop taking one of your herbs and see what happens. If you're still having a problem, stop taking that one and go back to the other—eventually (probably sooner rather than later) you'll figure it out.

Another option is using a combination herb supplement. Gastroenterologist at The Johns Hopkins Hospital Dr. Gerard Mullin and colleagues studied two regimens: Biotics Research FC-Cidal plus Biotics Research Dysbiocide, 2 caps twice a day for four weeks for each formula, or Metagenics Candibactin-AR with Metagenics Candibactin-BR, 2 caps twice a day for four weeks for each formula. They found that the herbal treatment was as effective as pharmaceutical antibiotics. However, as Dr. Siebecker points out, methane-SIBO patients will need to add allicin to the above regimes, and also the berberine dose in Candibactin-BR is fairly low and may need to be increased.

As with any condition requiring antibiotics—herbal or pharmaceutical—finding the right match and the right dose are the keys to success.

## The Elemental Diet (a.k.a. Starve the Suckers)

The elemental diet is a liquid medical food diet that consists of a specific mixture of predigested nutrients we need in order to live and comes either in a premixed liquid form or in powder form—in which case you need to mix it with water. The way it works is that these predigested nutrients are absorbed so quickly and so high up in the digestive tract that you get the same number of calories you would if you were eating regular food, but the bacteria in your small intestine are not being fed and, therefore, they starve to death. Other "shakes," meal replacements, and protein powders are not the same as the elemental diet (although you can use an elemental diet serving as a meal replacement, even if you're not following the elemental diet).

This is certainly the most difficult treatment method to follow, but it is also the fastest and, in many cases, it can decrease severe gas levels in a single two-week course. Some doctors will tell you it shouldn't be the first form of treatment, but others say it's been proven to work relatively quickly and effectively in most cases, so you might just decide to go for it before you've even tried one of the other two treatments.

One downside is that, because we associate eating so strongly with socializing, pleasure, and satisfaction, you might feel that, at least on an emotional level, you're starving to death along with the bacteria. But, on the other hand, some people report feeling so great on the diet that they say they wish they could stay on it forever.

Luckily, the elemental diet has come a long way in the very recent past. The original, unflavored version studied by Dr. Pimentel for SIBO, called Vivonex Plus, is made by Nestlé and doesn't taste good, but there are now several flavored formulas available that make it much more palatable.

## Elemental Diet Formulas with Flavor

Elemental Heal (whey-free) from Functional Medicine Formulations

https://store.drruscio.com/products/elemental-heal

Elemental Nutrition (Vanilla) and Keto-Elemental Nutrition from Vita Aid Professional Therapeutics (available only through a practitioner)

https://www.vitaaid.com/main/product.asp?ID=1160

https://www.vitaaid.com/usa/main/product.asp?ID=1160

Physicians' Elemental Diet and Physicians' Elemental Diet
Dextrose-Free from Integrative Therapeutics (available only
through a practitioner)
https://www.integrativepro.com/Products/Gastrointestinal
/Physicians-Elemental-Diet

Or, you can also make your own. For a "recipe," see https://www
.siboinfo.com/elemental-formula.html.

And really, if you know what the light is at the end of the tunnel, wouldn't you be willing to do almost anything for just two weeks—especially if it's going to give you the rest of your life back?

One potential problem I should mention is that the formula is necessarily high in simple carbohydrates because "elemental" means that the carbohydrate is broken down to its simplest form, which is glucose or maltodextrin depending on the formula. If you're someone who is susceptible to yeast, it could create some overgrowth. If you have a history of yeast, or certainly if you have an active yeast infection, you might want to talk to your doctor about taking some kind of antifungal, such as nystatin, which stays in the intestinal tract, along with the elemental formula.

Having changed your diet and completed at least one of the treatments for eliminating the overgrowth of bacteria in your small intestine, you should be well on your way to reclaiming your health and your life. If your case is complicated, as mine is, you may still be experiencing some symptoms or find yourself relapsing. But fear not: In the next chapter you'll learn what you can do to maintain or recover the progress you've already made.

To view the references cited in this chapter, please visit healingsibo.com/references.

# CHAPTER 7

# Retesting, Relapsing, Re-treating

Okay, you've been through your treatment protocol, you've been following the SIBO Specific Food Guide for at least three weeks, and, hopefully, you're experiencing relief from your symptoms.

What do you do now? The answer is, it depends, as is shown in the chart below.

I created this chart based on previous charts designed by Drs. Sie-becker and Sandberg-Lewis, which itself is a variation of Dr. Pimen-tel's IBS-SIBO chart.

## ARE YOU FEELING 90 PERCENT BETTER?

If you've completed treatment and are feeling 90 percent better or more, you don't need to retest. Woohoo! You can happily assume that your SIBO is resolved and you're now into a new phase: preventing relapse.

Relapse with SIBO is common, and if you do relapse, it's normal—but there are steps you can take starting immediately that will help you prevent it.

First, you should start a prokinetic right away. If you've been taking them all along, don't stop now. If you haven't been taking them, now's the time to start.

## ? SO YOU THINK YOU HAVE SIBO?

**SYMPTOMATIC RELIEF pg #45**

**DR. SIEBECKER'S SIBO SPECIFIC FOOD GUIDE pg #211**

**3-HOUR LACTULOSE BREATH TEST**

NEGATIVE → CONSIDER OTHER DIAGNOSES

POSITIVE → **CHOOSE A TREATMENT**

**ELEMENTAL DIET**

**HERBALS**
ALLICIN, NEEM & OREGANO pg #105

**ANTIBIOTICS**
RIFAXIMIN & NEOMYCIN pg #103

**TEST AGAIN**

**MANAGEMENT pg #109** ← NEGATIVE

POSITIVE → **TREAT AGAIN**

**PROKINETICS**  **DIET**

**INVESTIGATE UNDERLYING CAUSES**

---

1] Based on the Siebecker and Sandberg-Lewis Algorithm

2] Variation of the Cedars-Sinai Protocol

3] Pimentel M. A New IBS Solution: Bacteria - The Missing Link in Treating Irritable Bowel Syndrome. 1st ed. Sherman Oaks: Health Point Press, 2006 p90

4] Siebecker A, Sandberg-Lewis S. Small Intestine Bacterial Overgrowth: Often-Ignored Cause of Irritable Bowel Syndrome. Townsend Lett. 2013; (Feb/Mar). p85-91. http://www.townsendletter.com/FebMarch2013/ibs0213.html

For most people, SIBO is initially caused by a deficient migrating motor complex. Once you've gone through treatment and the bacteria have been cleared, or even partially cleared, you need to prevent them from coming back, and having a functional MMC is key. Prokinetics keep the MMC sweeping and help prevent other problems, such as acid reflux, that would allow what's been swept out to come back up.

Dr. Pimentel recommends taking prokinetics for three months after finishing treatment and then stopping on a trial basis to see how things go. For many people, that will be enough time, but some people with chronic cases will probably need to keep taking them permanently.

To revisit Dr. Siebecker's list of reliable prokinetics, see page 12.

Meal spacing is another way to support a healthy MMC and prevent relapse. The MMC runs on a ninety-minute cycle. If no calories (food or beverage) enter your body for ninety minutes, the MMC will do a sweep. Therefore, most doctors recommend three to four hours between meals to make sure the MMC has time to do its work. If you hear your stomach growling between meals, that's a good sign. It means the MMC is doing a sweep!

## IF YOU'RE NOT FEELING 90 PERCENT BETTER (YET)

If you've completed your first treatment (herbal antibiotics, antibiotics, or the elemental diet) and you're still not feeling at least 90 percent better than you did before changing your diet and starting treatment, if you would like to be able to expand your diet, or if you still have unresolved health issues, Drs. Siebecker and Sandberg-Lewis recommend you retest to see whether or not the SIBO is gone. The retesting should be done within two weeks of completing treatment because two-thirds of the people who have SIBO will relapse, many will relapse within two weeks, and the point of retesting is to see how effective your treatment was *before* you relapsed.

It could be that your first round of treatment didn't do the job.

Maybe it didn't work at all; maybe you saw only a slight improvement; or maybe you felt even worse. Personally, I was really let down when I finished my first round of rifaximin and still didn't feel well. Weren't the antibiotics supposed to cure me? I'd started the treatment with so much hope and excitement, and now I was really disappointed and felt somehow cheated. What was going on? I didn't know at the time that most of us will need more than one round of treatment.

If you've done the treatment and retested and found that your gas levels have gone down, congratulations, the treatment is working! You may still be positive for SIBO, but if your breath test numbers have come down even a little, you should consider your treatment a success; keep going! But if you initially tested positive for SIBO, were treated, and after your treatment protocol your gas levels didn't change, it might be time to try a different SIBO treatment. For example, if you were taking conventional antibiotics, perhaps you should try taking herbs. Or maybe it's time to move on to something more aggressive, such as the elemental diet.

The point is that if you don't feel at least 90 percent better, you need to get retested within two weeks because your SIBO might be gone even though you don't actually feel that much better, meaning something else was causing the symptoms. Or, you might have improved even though you don't feel much better yet. Or, if you haven't improved, you need to find out why. What you shouldn't do is panic. Just because your first treatment didn't work well doesn't mean you will feel this way forever.

## WHEN THE BACTERIA GO INTO HIDING

We tend to think of bacteria as individual organisms circulating in your intestinal tract, but they also form groups, and then hide out in what are called biofilms so that medications can't reach them.

The bacteria attach themselves to the lining of your intestine and secrete a mucous-like substance that forms a protective layer over them, making it difficult for the antibiotics you're taking to reach their intended target. I think of biofilms as an impenetrable tent the bacteria build to live inside.

We all have bacteria and we all have biofilms—it's normal. Things become problematic when we need to fight off bacterial infections. If you're taking antibiotics, it's normal for bacteria to want to reinforce their biofilm, because they want to survive as much as you want them to go away. So it can become an all-out war. According to the National Institutes of Health, almost 80 percent of human bacterial infections are associated with biofilms.

If you've been taking medication and you're still not getting better, you can try "biofilm busters." Once you are able to bust through the biofilm, your antibiotic medication should begin to work as it should and you will begin to see those formerly elusive results you've been looking for. Oregano, thyme, rosemary, volatile spices, curcumin, capsaicin, and olive leaf can help break up biofilms. And if those still don't do the trick, you can move on to more powerful treatments, which include:

- Interfase Plus by Klaire Labs
- Biofilm Phase-2 Advanced by Priority One

However, many doctors report mixed results using antibiofilm agents, which is why there isn't a standard SIBO recommended regimen. Personally, I think this is an area of great promise for the future.

## YOU MAY BE BETTER AND STILL FEEL BAD

If your gas level was very high, it might need to come down significantly before your symptoms are relieved. Therefore, retesting within two weeks will not only let you know where you are, it will also tell you how far you've come, and that can be very encouraging. Not re-testing is one of the biggest mistakes Dr. Siebecker sees, and she has tirelessly campaigned to shine a light on this blind spot.

On the breath test, a rise in hydrogen of more than 20 parts per million (of breath) or a rise in methane of more than 10 parts per million in ninety minutes is considered positive for SIBO, so if your initial level was extremely high, you may have come down a lot but still be positive for SIBO, even though you've actually made phenomenal progress. Remember, multiple rounds of treatment are usually needed, not just one (or two).

If you're at the end of your elemental diet treatment, you should test immediately after finishing. The elemental diet is done for two weeks, after which you need to fast overnight (for twelve hours) and retest on day fifteen, according to Dr. Pimentel. That's because there are some people who won't test negative after two weeks, but if those people stay on the diet for an additional week, they have a better chance to eradicate SIBO. Since the test results are almost immediate, they can continue the diet without losing any time. Otherwise they might have to start all over again, and no one wants to stay on the elemental diet any longer than is absolutely necessary. Be sure to plan in advance so that you have the kit on hand and communicate with the lab that you'll need the results within twenty-four hours.

Another important reason to retest is that SIBO is often associated with other conditions and diseases. If you don't feel better, or if you relapse quickly, it may be because you have some other, associated condition that needs to be checked out and dealt with. Some people (like me) have underlying causes that put them at greater risk of relapse. It isn't a life sentence, but it does require more maintenance.

According to Dr. Pimentel, "If you respond to rifaximin or an herbal antibiotic or some antibiotic and you're doing great, then getting to the bottom of it isn't so important, because, as I say, for 80 percent of patients it's the migrating motor complex. It's if the patient is relapsing really quickly that it's important to get to the bottom of it . . . if you took an antibiotic and you got better and it came back in a week, then you have to start thinking about things that are causing the SIBO."

If you do test negative once you've completed your treatment, but you still have symptoms, you need to start looking for other problems. According to Dr. Siebecker, SIBO is common in people who have autoimmune diseases such as IBD, scleroderma, celiac disease, and Hashimoto's hypothyroidism, although the exact nature of these associations isn't fully known. However, because increased intestinal permeability (that is, leaky gut)—along with a genetic susceptibility and exposure to a trigger (such as Cdt-B with food poisoning)—is one of the three underlying causes of autoimmunity, "SIBO, with its high likelihood of generating leaky gut, will need to be corrected for both prevention and treatment of autoimmunity," she says.

What about if you still test positive but are feeling better? One of the tricky things about SIBO is that the amount of bacteria you have doesn't always correlate with the severity of your symptoms. That means your gas levels could be very high on a test, but you feel good, while another person could have only slightly elevated levels and horrible symptoms. For some people, a negative SIBO breath test is the ultimate goal, and they are willing to continue treatment until they get there. Other people are happy to feel 90 percent better, even if they still have some level of SIBO. That leads many people to assume that if they are feeling good, they don't need to retest, but it's not that black and white. It's also possible that you don't have SIBO anymore, and symptoms are caused by something else. That's why it is always a good idea to retest after treatment.

## UNDERLYING CAUSES AND ASSOCIATED DISEASES

Other diseases associated with SIBO include Crohn's disease, hypothyroid, and diabetes, all of which are very common. Ehlers-Danlos, a group of connective tissue disorders, is not as rare as one might think.

In fact, 60 percent of those with constipation-type IBS and 35 percent of those with diarrhea-type IBS have Ehlers-Danlos. And then there's Parkinson's; scleroderma; POTS (postural orthostatic tachycardia syndrome), a condition that affects circulation; and injuries such as traumatic brain injury (which could actually result from nothing more than falling off your bicycle), traumatic spinal injury, or whiplash, any of which can be caused by a car accident.

It might seem crazy to think that an injury to your head could somehow cause bacterial overgrowth, but it actually makes sense when you consider that your brain and your gut are in direct communication with each other through the vagus nerve.

The vagus nerve controls the function of the migrating motor complex, and when you experience a traumatic brain injury, proper communication between the vagus nerve and the migrating motor complex can be impacted, which can create a situation in which SIBO can develop.

Other associated conditions to be aware of, according to Dr. Siebecker:

- Inadequate bile acids
- Low stomach acid
- Low pancreatic enzymes
- Stress (which can impact motility)
- Diverticulitis
- Liver disease
- Restless leg syndrome
- Chronic renal failure
- Post-chemotherapy
- Rheumatoid arthritis
- Interstitial cystitis

## What Is POTS?

You may never have heard of it, but that doesn't mean you might not have it. Postural orthostatic tachycardia syndrome occurs when your vagus nerve isn't functioning properly and therefore your sympathetic nervous system is working in overdrive. This not only impacts your digestion but also affects your ability to move from a reclining to a standing position. Your heart rate shoots up and you get light-headed but you don't faint. If you experience that phenomenon on a regular basis, you may have POTS, which could also be causing your SIBO symptoms because you're not in "rest and digest" mode.

The important thing for you to consider is that if you have symptoms of POTS, the POTS may be an underlying cause of your SIBO. A doctor can do a simple test by taking your pulse when you're lying down and again when you stand up to confirm that you have the condition.

A good way to think of it is that SIBO is really a symptom that has its own symptoms and issues. SIBO doesn't happen on its own. This is important to understand. Imagine that you had a faucet leaking water onto the floor. SIBO is like the water on the floor. Yes, you need to clean it up, but if you don't also fix the plumbing, you'll be cleaning water off the floor forever.

## SIBO and Lyme Disease—the Gut-Brain Connection

Commonly associated with tick bites, Lyme disease is technically an infection caused by the spirochete *Borrelia burgdorferi* (and, no, you New Yorkers, that's not a place you go on a shopping spree), which can cause both gastrointestinal and neurological problems similar to SIBO. In other words, Lyme can either cause or contribute to a person's SIBO symptoms. If your SIBO is cleared but your symptoms persist, it would, therefore, be a good idea to get tested for Lyme disease. Lyme Disease expert Dr. Tom Messinger recommends the at-home Lyme test from DNA Connexions.

You need to keep looking for that underlying cause, because if you treat the bacterial overgrowth without treating whatever interfered with the proper functioning of the MMC or caused your motility issues in the first place, you're not going to be able to treat SIBO successfully. Some underlying causes can be resolved and some will need to be managed for life. But at least you will know what to do in order to manage your SIBO. And your life can still be 100 percent better with a managed chronic condition than with one that is unmanaged.

## FINDING THE ROOT CAUSE

Sometimes the cause of SIBO is obvious and sometimes it isn't. In many cases, you have SIBO but you also have other health problems that are probably not what caused your SIBO. Both fibromyalgia and rosacea patients, for example, have been shown to have higher than normal levels of hydrogen gas (and in the case of rosacea, sometimes also methane) on the lactulose breath test. Fibromyalgia is a condition causing widespread musculoskeletal pain as well as fatigue, brain fog, and sleep issues. Rosacea is a condition in which the skin of the face becomes red and blotchy. In the fibromyalgia patients, a higher gas level correlated with a higher pain level, and in another study, fibromyalgia sufferers were shown to have an increased prevalence of leaky gut. When the rosacea patients were treated with antibiotics for either the hydrogen or methane gas, the vast majority saw a significant decrease or complete remission of symptoms. It seems clear that there is a relationship between these two conditions and SIBO. But exactly what that relationship is remains unknown—at least for the moment.

At a certain point, however, it really doesn't matter which came first or how your health issues are related. You've got them both and you have to address them in order to have the best outcome you can.

## Beauty from the Inside Out

In addition to rosacea, psoriasis, eczema, and acne often accompany SIBO. For years these conditions have been treated mainly with antibiotic creams, but, in fact, while topical treatments do help, these skin problems often have deeper causes, and to clear them up once and for all, you need to find and treat the underlying cause.

## OTHER HEALTH ISSUES THAT MIMIC SIBO

In addition to being associated with other health problems, SIBO symptoms can also mimic a whole host of other diseases. Some of them may be less of a problem, while others can be serious. Bloating, for example, is a symptom of ovarian cancer as well as a temporary response to eating beans or cruciferous vegetables, but don't start jumping to conclusions or catastrophizing (like I so often did). Chances are you just have a complicated case of SIBO, but better safe than sorry, as they say. So if you are still not better after treating your SIBO, here is an alphabetical list of other health issues from Dr. Siebecker that often have similar symptoms:

Bile acid malabsorption

Cancer

Celiac Disease

Endometriosis

Food intolerances

Fructose intolerance

Gastroparesis

Gut dysbiosis/large intestine bacterial overgrowth

*Helicobacter pylori* (*H. pylori*)

Histamine intolerance

Hypo- or hyperthyroid

Hypochloridia (low stomach acid)

Immune deficiency

Inflammatory bowel disease (Crohn's or ulcerative colitis)

Insufficient chewing

Lactose intolerance

Pancreatic enzyme insufficiency

Parasite infection

Salicylate intolerance

Small intestine obstruction

Stress

Yeast overgrowth (Candida)

To view the references cited in this chapter, please visit healingsibo.com/references.

# CHAPTER 8

# SIBO-Friendly Recipes

Although I follow Dr. Siebecker's SIBO Specific Food Guide, some of you may already be following one of the other SIBO diet plans. So again, at the beginning of each recipe I've indicated the other diets for which they would be appropriate. Here is a guide to each label:

**BPD: Bi-Phasic Diet**
**SCD: Specific Carbohydrate Diet**
**LF: Low FODMAP Diet**
**CSD: Cedars-Sinai Low Fermentation Diet**
**SSFG: SIBO Specific Food Guide**

When you see SSFG★, the asterisk indicates that the recipe contains one or more ingredients—such as gluten-free bread or potato—that are not in the SIBO Specific Food Guide but are in other SIBO diets and are tolerated by many people with SIBO. So if you tolerate that ingredient, you can include it in the recipe.

And, just as a reminder, I'm a vegetarian, as are all of the recipes in this chapter. If you wish, you can add a protein of your choice from those listed on page 217.

Finally, in certain instances throughout these recipes I call for an ingredient—mustard or ketchup, for example—that is "SIBO-friendly."

What I mean by that is simply that you use a variety or brand of this ingredient that doesn't contain anything that would be irritating to people with SIBO (garlic, onion, or dairy that contains lactose). Common ingredients to look out for are gums or thickeners like carrageenan and guar gum, which are often in nondairy milks, yogurt, ice cream, sauces, and condiments. See the red foods in the SIBO Specific Food Guide (Appendix, page 211) and check the label before you buy!

All of these recipes are easy to prepare, most of them are quick and tasty, so you won't feel "SIBO deprived."

## RECIPE GROCERY LIST

Here is a list of essential ingredients to stock up on before you begin the 21-Day plan.

### Pantry Items
- Almond flour
- Artichoke hearts, canned
- Baking soda
- Butter
- Chia seeds
- Chocolate chips, dark & dairy-free (as tolerated)
- Coconut: flakes, flour, and shredded
- Coconut aminos
- Coconut milk, full fat (without gums)
- Cranberries, dried
- Dried herbs and spices: Bay leaves; black pepper: freshly ground, black peppercorns, whole; cayenne pepper; chili flakes; cinnamon; coriander: seeds and ground; cumin; fennel; five spice; ginger; Italian herbs (without garlic); lavender (culinary grade); mustard, ground; nutmeg; paprika; thyme
- Earl Grey tea

- Espresso or coffee
- Ghee
- Honey (clover—filtered, not raw)
- Kalamata olives
- Lentils, canned
- Mustard, prepared (SIBO-friendly)
- Oils: avocado, coconut, garlic, MCT, olive, walnut
- Pumpkin
- Relish (SIBO-friendly)
- Rice and rice products: brown or white (short- or medium-grain), rice cakes, wraps
- Salsa (SIBO-friendly)
- Sea salt
- Tomato paste (organic)
- Tomato sauce (organic, tomatoes only)
- Vanilla extract
- Vegetable broth powder
- Vinegars: apple cider, champagne, rice wine (without sugar), white wine vinegar
- Yogurt starter

**Refrigerator Items:**
- Almond butter
- Butter
- Cheese: Cheddar, mild (aged 30 days or more); Gruyère; Parmesan
- Eggs (pasture raised and organic if possible)
- Hot sauce (SIBO-friendly)
- Maple syrup
- Mayonnaise (SIBO-friendly)
- Milk: SIBO-friendly milk of choice, whole 100% lactose-free dairy milk

- Nuts: almonds (raw slivered), pecans (raw pieces), pumpkin seeds (raw), walnuts (raw pieces)
- Strawberries, organic

### Garlic Oil

I love to cook with garlic oil. It provides delicious flavor without adding high FODMAPs because you don't eat the actual garlic's fermentable fiber. You can use store-bought garlic oil or, to make it yourself, cut a garlic clove in half and sauté it in olive oil. Then remove and discard the garlic clove and use the oil immediately.

**Produce:**
- Arugula
- Avocado
- Bananas
- Bell peppers (green, red, and yellow)
- Blueberries (fresh or frozen)
- Broccoli
- Cabbage, red or purple
- Carrots
- Celery
- Citrus fruits: grapefruit, lemons, limes, oranges, tangerines (organic for zesting)
- English cucumbers
- Green onion
- Ginger
- Herbs: basil, chives, cilantro, dill, mint, parsley, rosemary, tarragon, thyme
- Lettuce (butter or red)
- Microgreens

- Pineapple
- Potatoes, russet and Yukon Gold (organic)
- Spinach (organic)
- Squash: delicata squash, spaghetti squash, zucchini
- Tomatoes (organic)

**Freezer Items:**
- Acai puree

## KITCHEN TOOLS LIST

These tools will make recipe preparation at home much simpler.

- Aluminum foil
- Baking sheets: 8-inch-square, 8 x 12-inch, or 9 x 12-inch baking sheet
- Blender
- Can opener
- Candy thermometer
- Chopsticks or Popsicle sticks
- Citrus juicer
- Cutting board
- Food processor
- Grater
- Hand mixer
- Ice cube tray
- Immersion blender
- Juicer
- Ladle
- Mason jars and other storage containers
- Measuring cups (for both wet and dry ingredients)
- Measuring spoons
- Mixing bowls (small, medium, and large)
- Muffin tin, 12-cup (silicon or traditional)

- Parchment paper
- Pastry brush
- Pie pan, 9-inch
- Pitcher
- Pots and pans (a variety of sizes, including saucepans and sauté pans, a soup pot, and a 10-inch ovenproof pan)
- Sharp knives
- Sieve or strainer (fine-mesh and general strainer)
- Vegetable peeler
- Whisks (large and small)
- Wooden spoons
- Yogurt maker
- Zester (for citrus)

# DRINKS

# Get Going Green Juice

### Dairy-free, Gluten-free, Nut-free, Egg-free
### Diets: LF, SCD, SSFG

---

**Serves 1 (approximately 1¼ cups juice)**
**Prep Time: 10 minutes**

Juicing is great for some people following a SIBO diet, but not for others. This juice, with its light sweetness and combination of healthy SIBO-friendly veggies, gets me going in the morning. You don't need to peel the vegetables, since you'll be juicing them and won't be digesting the fiber. You will need a juicer to prepare this recipe. Buy organic fruits and vegetables whenever possible.

½ cup chopped green bell pepper
½ English cucumber, chopped
1 carrot, chopped
½ cup fresh or canned (in juice, not syrup) pineapple
1-inch piece of ginger
1 cup (packed) fresh greens, such as arugula or organic spinach

Put all of the ingredients into the juicer and process. Pour the juice into your glass and enjoy immediately. If you're very sensitive, you might want to strain the juice again.

**Note:**
This juice will keep in the refrigerator for approximately 2 days, but I think it tastes best when it's freshly made.

# Refreshing Basil-Cucumber Water

Dairy-free, Gluten-free, Nut-free, Egg-Free

Diets: BPD—Phase I, LF, SCD, SSFG

---

**Serves 4**

**Prep Time: 10 minutes**

Having flavored water available often gets us to drink more. Many health practitioners recommend that you drink half your body weight in ounces each day. So if you weigh 150 pounds, you should be drinking at least 75 ounces of water a day. This turns a beautiful emerald color when blended, but if you prefer, or if you don't have a blender, you can add the cucumber and basil to the water without blending it. If you do that, just make sure to use a pitcher with a stopper so the cucumber and basil don't get poured into your glass, because they will probably get mushy and not taste so good.

1 medium cucumber, peeled, seeded, and chopped or 1 English
   cucumber, peeled and chopped
¼ cup freshly squeezed lime juice
Zest of 1 organic lime
½ cup chopped basil

Measure 4 cups of cold water into your blender container. Add the cucumber, lime juice, zest, and basil and blend for approximately 1 minute or until the mixture is smooth.

Strain the mixture into a pitcher to remove any pulp.

Serve immediately over ice or refrigerate and enjoy for up to 1 week.

**Variation:**

Try making this water with orange, mint, lemon, or other flavors you love.

# Nutty Ginger Banana Smoothie

**Dairy-free, Gluten-free, Egg-free**

**Diets: CSD, LF, SCD, SSFG**

---

**Serves 1**

**Prep Time: 5 minutes**

This is a simple-to-make yet satisfying smoothie that will get your day started right. If you want a bigger protein boost, you can add the protein powder of your choice. If you tolerate cocoa, you can add a tablespoon for a chocolatey flavor. If you love ginger, you can add even more.

2 tablespoons almond butter (or another nut butter of your choice)
1 tablespoon peeled and chopped fresh ginger
1 medium frozen banana
¾ cup SIBO-friendly milk of your choice
1 teaspoon MCT oil (see Note)

Place the almond butter, ginger, banana, milk, and MCT oil in a blender. Blend for 1 minute or until all of the ingredients are liquefied, and serve immediately.

**Note:**

MCT oil is a supplement made from medium-chain triglycerides, which are easy to digest due to the shorter length of the triglyceride chain. Because of that, they act as an immediate source of energy. If you are not used to consuming MCT oil, start with 1 teaspoon and work up to the full tablespoon called for in the recipe.

# Honey Lavender Latte

**Dairy-free, Gluten-free**

**Diets: BPD—Phase I, CSD, LF, SCD, SSFG**

---

**Serves I**

**Prep Time: 5 minutes**

Even though lavender is floral, it has a surprisingly delicious taste
when combined with honey in this latte. It's a perfect drink in any
season. To me this is like a yoga retreat in a mug.

1 cup SIBO-friendly milk of choice, heated
½ cup hot espresso or other strong coffee
1 tablespoon Lavender Simple Syrup (page 207)

Froth the milk by using a hand frother, if you have one, or shake it in
a covered jar until frothy.

Pour the coffee into a mug large enough to accommodate the
milk. Stir in the simple syrup and the frothed milk.

Serve immediately.

**Cooking Tip:**
You can vary the amount of each ingredient to find the ratio that is
just right for you.

# Earl Grey Latte

Dairy-free, Gluten-free, Nut-free, Egg-free

Diets: BPD—Phase I, CSD, SCD, SSFG

---

**Serves I**

**Cook Time: I0**

This latte makes a delicious and unique morning beverage. You can make it in larger batches, store it in the refrigerator, and warm a cup whenever you want. You can also drink it iced if you prefer.

1 bag Earl Grey tea

1 cup boiling water

1 tablespoon Lavender Simple Syrup (page 207)

1 teaspoon vanilla extract

½ cup SIBO-friendly milk of your choice, heated

Place the tea bag in a cup and cover with the boiling water. Let steep for 3 to 5 minutes before removing the tea bag.

Add the simple syrup and vanilla to the hot tea and stir.

Froth the milk with a hand frother, if you have one, or shake it in a covered jar until frothy.

Stir the frothed milk into the tea and serve immediately.

**Cooking Tip:**

You can add more or less milk and/or simple syrup to suit your personal taste.

# BREAKFASTS

# Blueberry-Lemon Muffins

### Dairy-free, Gluten-free
### Diets: LF, SCD, SSFG

---

**Serves 12 (1 muffin per serving)**
Prep Time: 10 minutes/Cook Time: 25 minutes

Thank goodness I can still have muffins even though I have SIBO.
These don't rise as much as muffins made with wheat flour, but
they're still delicious. They will keep, tightly covered, in the
refrigerator for up to 1 week, and they can also be frozen. Remove
from the freezer and warm in the oven or the microwave for
breakfast or a snack.

2 cups almond flour
¾ teaspoon baking soda
½ teaspoon sea salt
2 large eggs
¼ cup clover honey
1 tablespoon plus 1 teaspoon olive oil
1 teaspoon vanilla extract
Zest of one organic lemon
2 tablespoons freshly squeezed lemon juice
1 cup blueberries, fresh or frozen

Preheat the oven to 350°F. Line a 12-cup muffin tin with silicon or
paper cups.

Place the almond flour, baking soda, and salt in a medium bowl
and stir until the ingredients are incorporated.

Add the eggs, honey, olive oil, vanilla, lemon zest, and lemon
juice to the dry ingredients and mix until well combined. Gently fold
in the blueberries.

Fill each muffin cup three-quarters full and bake for 20 to 25 minutes or until the muffins are golden brown.

Remove from the oven and cool for 5 minutes before removing the muffins from the tin.

**Variations:**

If you don't like or can't tolerate blueberries, you can substitute another type of berry. You can also replace the lemon zest and juice with orange zest and juice, which are slightly sweeter.

**Ingredient Tip:**

When you're buying honey, make sure that it's actually certified honey, and that it's cooked, doesn't have the comb in it, and doesn't have added ingredients, such as high-fructose corn syrup.

# Easy Veggie Scramble

Gluten-free, Nut-free

Diets: BPD, CSD, LF, SCD, SSFG

---

**Serves: I**

Prep Time: 5 minutes/Cook Time: 7 minutes

The beauty of a veggie scramble is that you can add whatever vegetables agree with you at any given time. Always start with the ones that take longest to cook and then add those with shorter cooking times. Last, add the eggs—easy peasy!

1 tablespoon butter, salted or unsalted or ghee, or coconut or avocado oil

¼ cup green, red, or yellow bell peppers, chopped into bite-size pieces

¼ cup broccoli florets, chopped into bite-size pieces

1 green onion (green part only), sliced

½ cup chopped arugula

2 large eggs, whisked

¼ cup shredded Cheddar cheese or other SIBO-friendly cheese of choice (optional)

Sea salt and freshly ground black pepper to taste

Melt the butter in a medium nonstick skillet over medium–high heat.

Add the bell pepper and broccoli and sauté for 2 minutes or until the vegetables turn golden and begin to soften.

Reduce the heat to medium and add the green onion and arugula. Cook for 2 more minutes.

Add the eggs and cheese if using and stir the mixture with a spatula as the eggs begin to cook. Add the salt and pepper and continue to stir until the eggs are cooked but not brown.

Remove from the heat and serve immediately.

**SIBO Tip:**

If you're having trouble keeping weight on, add a second tablespoon of ghee, butter, or oil to the scramble when you add in the eggs. It will make the scramble extra rich and also add some calories.

# 24-Hour Yogurt

**Gluten-free, Nut-free, Egg-free**

**Diets: BPD, LF, SCD, SSFG**

---

**Serves 8**

**Prep Time: 30 minutes/Cook Time: 24 hours**

Making your own yogurt can seem daunting, but once you've done it once or twice you'll realize how easy it is. Topped with honey, granola, or fruit, this is a great breakfast. And the yogurt can also be used in many recipes, including smoothies or the Ranch Dressing recipe on page 187.

Cooking the yogurt for 24 hours removes all the lactose, making it low fermentable and a probiotic powerhouse. For many people, 24-Hour Yogurt is a supportive part of their diet because it helps them maintain weight or have better bowel movements. Start with a small amount (such as a teaspoon or a tablespoon) and start increasing the quantity to determine your own tolerance level.

## Special Equipment:

YOGURT MAKER

CANDY THERMOMETER

2 quarts whole milk or half-and-half (or amount as specified on
    your yogurt maker)
1 packet Yogourmet yogurt starter or another SIBO-friendly
    starter of your choice

Make an ice water bath by placing two trays of ice cubes and cold water in a pan large enough to hold the saucepan you will use to heat the milk.

Place the milk in a medium saucepan over medium-high heat. Attach the thermometer to the side of the pan and heat the milk to 180°F, stirring frequently.

Place the pan in the ice water bath until the milk cools to 110°F, stirring frequently.

Add ½ cup of the cooled milk to the yogurt machine container. Add the yogurt starter and whisk to combine thoroughly with the milk. Whisk in the rest of the milk and place the top on the yogurt container.

Heat at 110 degrees for 24 hours, then refrigerate for about 3 hours until firm.

## Acai Smoothie Bowl

### Dairy-free, Gluten-free, Nut-free, Egg-free

### Diets: CSD, LF, SCD, SSFG

---

**Serves 1**

**Prep Time: 10 minutes**

I love beautiful and nutrient-dense smoothie bowls! Plus, they taste just as good as ice cream.

One 100-gram package frozen acai puree, defrosted
1 frozen banana
¼ cup frozen blueberries
⅛ cup SIBO friendly milk of your choice, or more as needed
¼ cup Grain-Free Granola (recipe follows) (optional)
1 tablespoon clover honey (optional)
Sliced fruit from SSFG green foods list on page 212 (optional)

Place the acai, banana, blueberries, and milk in a blender and process until smooth.

If the mixture is too thick and isn't blending well, add in another tablespoon of milk.

Pour the mixture into a bowl and top with granola if using, honey if desired, fruit if using, or another topping of your choice and serve immediately.

# Berry Compote

**Dairy-free, Gluten-free, Nut-free, Egg-free**

**Diets: BPD, CSD, LF, SCD, SSFG**

---

**Makes about 3 cups**

**Prep Time: 5 minutes/Cook Time: 20 minutes**

If you use strawberries in this recipe, consider buying organic because the Environmental Working Group (EWG) lists strawberries among the Dirty Dozen—that is, one of the fruits with the most pesticide residue when conventionally grown.

2 tablespoons coconut oil, salted or unsalted butter, or ghee
4 cups blueberries and/or organic strawberries, fresh or frozen
2 teaspoons freshly squeezed lemon juice (optional)
1 tablespoon clover honey (optional)

Place the oil in a medium saucepan over medium heat. When it is melted, add the fruit, lemon juice if using, and honey if desired and stir to combine.

Bring to a simmer, stirring occasionally, and reduce the heat to medium-low. Cook for about 20 minutes, stirring occasionally, until the mixture thickens to your liking.

Serve immediately or store tightly covered in the refrigerator for up to 1 week.

**Cooking Tip:**
For a thicker compote, cook the berries a bit longer. For a thinner compote, reduce the cooking time. The berries can also be blended with an immersion blender to break them down and make them more digestible.

# Grain-Free Granola

### Dairy-free, Gluten-free, Egg-free
### Diets: BPD, CSD, LF, SCD, SSFG

---

**Serves 8 (½-cup serving)**
**Prep Time: 5 minutes/Cook Time: 20 minutes**

This granola is also good as a breakfast cereal and makes an excellent topping for yogurt. Nuts and coconut can be hard for some people to digest, so start with a smaller amount if you're not sure of your tolerance.

⅔ cup unsweetened coconut flakes (not shredded coconut)
1 cup raw slivered almonds
1¼ cups raw pecan pieces
1¼ cups raw walnut pieces
½ cup raw pepitas (hulled pumpkin seeds)
3 tablespoons chia seeds (optional; don't use for BPD, SCD, SSFG)
⅓ cup dried cranberries
1 teaspoon five spice powder
½ teaspoon sea salt
2 tablespoons olive oil or melted coconut oil
¼ cup maple syrup
1 teaspoon vanilla extract

Preheat the oven to 350°F. Line a rimmed baking sheet with parchment paper or aluminum foil.

Place the coconut flakes, almonds, pecans, walnuts, pepitas, chia seeds, and cranberries on the prepared baking sheet.

In a small bowl, mix the five spice powder, salt, oil, maple syrup, and vanilla.

Pour the spice mixture over the nuts and stir to make sure all the nuts are coated. Spread the nuts out on the baking sheet and bake for about 9 minutes.

Remove from the oven, stir, and bake for 9 more minutes. Cool completely on the baking sheet set on a wire rack.

The granola will keep at room temperature in an airtight container for about 2 weeks.

**Ingredient Note:**
If you don't like five spice powder, feel free to replace it with cinnamon or just leave it out. You can also use different kinds of nuts, depending on your preference.

# Frozen Blueberry Yogurt Bites

Gluten-free, Nut-free optional, Egg-free

Diets: BPD, CSD, LF, SCD, SSFG

---

**Makes 12 large or 24 small bites**

Prep Time: 10 minutes/Cook Time: 5 minutes

Now you can have delicious frozen yogurt with granola on the go! Leave out the grain-free granola to make the recipe nut-free. You can also use a different type of fruit if you prefer.

1 cup fresh or frozen and defrosted blueberries

2 tablespoons clover honey

1 cup full-fat 24-Hour Yogurt (page 138)

1 cup Grain-Free Granola (page 142) (optional)

Place a full-size 12-cup silicone muffin tin or a 24-cup miniature-size silicon muffin tin on a baking sheet.

Combine the blueberries and honey in a medium bowl.

Crush the blueberries with the back of a wooden spoon until at least half are broken and juicy.

Add the 24-Hour Yogurt and mix well.

Divide the granola equally among the muffin cups.

Spoon the yogurt mixture over the granola and freeze for 2 or more hours.

Store in a glass or plastic container in the freezer.

**Ingredient Tip:**

The ingredients in this recipe are breakfast foods, but you can make these frozen yogurt treats into a dessert by adding more honey, some dairy-free chocolate chips, or any other delicious items you can tolerate.

# APPETIZERS AND SNACKS

## Angel Eggs

Dairy-free, Gluten-free, Nut-free

Diets: BPD, CSD, LF, SCD, SSFG

---

**Serves 12 (2 per serving)**

Prep Time: 15 minutes/Cook Time: 15 to 20 minutes

if you're boiling your own eggs

These are called "Deviled Eggs," but I like a more positive name. If you're not cooking for a crowd, you can halve this recipe. Organic or cage-free hard-boiled eggs are also at many stores, including Costco and Trader Joe's.

12 large hard-boiled eggs

⅓ cup nondairy SIBO-friendly mayonnaise

1 tablespoon plus 1 teaspoon SIBO-friendly mustard

2 shakes SIBO-friendly hot sauce, such as McIlhenny Tabasco (optional)

½ teaspoon sea salt

Paprika for garnish (optional)

Cut each egg in half lengthwise and separate the yolks from the whites, being careful to keep the whites in one piece.

Place the yolks in a medium bowl and the whites on a platter.

Crumble the yolks with a fork and add the mayonnaise, mustard, hot sauce if using, and salt.

Mix well. If the mixture is too thick for your particular taste, add more mayonnaise or mustard until it is the consistency and flavor you prefer.

Place 1 teaspoon of the yolk mixture into the center of each egg white. Garnish with paprika if desired and serve immediately.

**Variations:**

Try adding herbs such as parsley or dill or using an additional topping such as Tapenade (page 206).

# Quick Pickled Cucumbers and Carrots

**Dairy-free, Gluten-free, Nut-free, Egg-free**

**Diets: BPD, CSD, LF, SCD, SSFG**

---

**Makes 12 to 16 ounces, about 12 servings**

**Prep Time: 10 minutes/Cook Time: 10 minutes**

**plus 24 hours refrigeration time**

You can do all carrots or all cucumbers for this recipe, if you prefer. And if you don't have time to make the pickles, you can eat the sliced cucumber dipped in rice wine vinegar. The pickled vegetables will keep for up to 4 weeks in the refrigerator.

1 English cucumber, cut into spears

2 carrots

1 cup clover honey

1 cup apple cider vinegar

1 cup white or sugar-free rice wine vinegar

1 tablespoon sea salt

1 tablespoon coriander seed

1 sprig fresh dill

½ teaspoon dry mustard

1 teaspoon whole black peppercorns

2 dried bay leaves, crumbled

1 pinch chili flakes (optional)

Place the cucumber spears in a quart-size Mason jar that will withstand boiling liquids. Place the carrots in an 8-ounce Mason jar.

Place the honey, vinegars, salt, coriander seed, dill, mustard, peppercorns, bay leaves, and chili flakes if using in a saucepan over medium-high heat.

Bring the mixture to boil, stirring frequently to incorporate the honey.

Remove from the heat and carefully pour the mixture over the cucumber and carrots.

Cool to room temperature, then cover and refrigerate for 24 hours.

**SIBO Tip:**
English cucumbers have thinner peels than regular cucumbers, but if you have difficulty digesting any foods with peels it's better to peel the cucumber.

# Roasted Artichoke Hearts

### Dairy-free, Gluten-free, Nut-free, Egg-free

### Diets: BPD, CSD, LF, SSFG*

---

**Serves 4**

**Prep Time: 5 minutes/Cook Time: 20 minutes**

These roasted artichoke hearts are delicious on their own, but you can also add them to a salad or use them for scooping up a dip, such as the Creamy Spinach Artichoke Dip (page 154).

One 14-ounce can water-packed artichoke hearts
1 tablespoon infused garlic oil (see page 124)
Sea salt and freshly ground black pepper to taste

Preheat the oven to 400°F. Line a rimmed baking sheet with
  parchment paper.
Drain the artichokes and squeeze any additional water from each
  one individually.
Cut the artichokes in half and place them in a medium mixing
  bowl with the garlic oil. Mix until the oil is evenly distributed.
  Sprinkle with salt and pepper and mix again.
Spread the artichokes cut-side down on the prepared baking sheet
  and bake for 20 minutes or until golden brown.

### SIBO Tip:

Normally, globe artichokes are high FODMAP, but because these are canned, the FODMAPs leech out into the water, which is discarded. This is typical of several higher FODMAP canned foods such as lentils.

*There is an asterisk following SSFG at the beginning of this recipe because canned vegetables are "red" foods on the SSFG (and illegal on the SCD). But that's because they may contain trace amounts of ingredients (less than 2 percent) that are not required to be listed on the label. I don't believe that most SIBO patients need to be quite that vigilant, and, in any case, I would never cook a fresh artichoke for myself, so if I want an artichoke in my life, canned or jarred is the way I go.

# Zesty Zucchini Pizza Bites

Gluten-free, Nut-free, Egg-free

Diets: BPD, LF, SCD, SSFG

---

**Serves 4 to 6**

Prep Time: I5 minutes/Cook Time: I5 minutes

If you don't like or tolerate tomato sauce, you can always top these with pesto instead. If fresh basil isn't available, try using another vegetable topping such as finely chopped bell pepper.

2 small to medium zucchini (½ to 1 pound total)

¾ teaspoon sea salt

⅛ cup SIBO-friendly organic tomato sauce (tomatoes only, such as Pomi), or more as needed

½ teaspoon dried Italian herb blend

2½ tablespoons garlic oil (see page 124)

⅓ cup grated Cheddar cheese (or other SIBO-friendly cheese of your choice), or more as needed

¼ cup chopped fresh basil (optional)

Preheat the oven to 400°F. Line a baking sheet large enough to hold all of the zucchini with parchment paper.

Cut the zucchini on the bias into ¼-inch-thick slices.

Place the zucchini slices in a colander, sprinkle with ½ teaspoon of the salt, and mix to coat all of the zucchini with the salt. Set aside for 10 minutes.

While the zucchini is draining, place the tomato sauce in a small saucepan and add the herbs, the remaining ¼ teaspoon of salt, and 1 tablespoon of the garlic oil.

Place over medium heat until the sauce is bubbling, then reduce the heat to low.

Place the remaining 1½ tablespoons of garlic oil in a small bowl.

Gently press the zucchini slices between two paper towels to remove any excess moisture.

With a pastry brush, brush the slices on both sides with the garlic oil and spread them on the prepared baking sheet in a single layer.

Bake in the preheated oven for 5 minutes. Remove from the oven but do not turn it off.

Carefully spoon approximately 1 teaspoon of sauce onto each slice and top with 1 teaspoon of the cheese. You may need more or less of both the tomato sauce and the cheese depending on the size of your zucchini.

Sprinkle a pinch of basil, if desired, over the cheese. Return to the oven for 10 minutes or until the cheese is melted.

Serve immediately.

**SIBO Tip:**

On the SCD diet, only hard aged cheese is considered "legal" because it is considered the only kind that is lactose free. However, according to the Monash University low FODMAP app, most cheese, in specified amounts, is low FODMAP and doesn't contain lactose. Another way to see if your cheese contains lactose is to look at the label. If it says 0 grams of sugar, that means it doesn't contain lactose, which is a fermentable milk sugar. That said, no matter which diet you're on, it's always important to test new foods in small amounts to see what you personally can tolerate.

# Creamy Spinach Artichoke Dip

### Gluten-free, Nut-free

### Diets: BPD, LF, SCD, SSFG

---

### Serves 8

### Prep Time: 5 minutes/Cook Time: 20 minutes

Creamy spinach dip is a perennial favorite. Here, we've just tweaked the ingredients to make it SIBO-friendly. You can scoop up the dip with SIBO-friendly crackers, vegetables, or the Roasted Artichoke Hearts (page 150).

1 cup chopped fresh organic spinach

One 14-ounce can water-packed artichoke hearts, drained and
    chopped

1 cup SIBO-friendly mayonnaise

1 cup freshly grated Parmesan cheese

1 tablespoon freshly squeezed lemon juice

Preheat the oven to 375°F.

In a medium bowl, combine the spinach, artichoke hearts, mayonnaise, cheese, and lemon juice.

Spread the mixture evenly in an 8-inch-square pan or a comparable casserole dish and bake in the preheated oven for 25 minutes or until golden brown. It may take 2 or 3 minutes longer.

### SIBO Tip:

While all of the ingredients in this dip are SIBO-friendly, the mayonnaise and Parmesan cheese make it quite heavy. If you have a problem absorbing fat, start with a small amount and see how you tolerate it.

# SOUPS, SALADS, AND SANDWICHES

# Broccoli Cheddar Soup

Gluten-free, Nut-free, Egg-free

Diets: BPD, LF, SCD, SSFG

---

**Serves 4**

Prep Time: 15 minutes/Cook Time: 30 minutes

Even though there is no cream in this soup, it has a depth of flavor, and both the broccoli and the Cheddar shine through. Freeze or store tightly covered in the refrigerator for up to 4 days.

2 tablespoons avocado oil

1 bunch green onions (green part only), chopped

1 stalk celery, chopped

2 carrots, chopped

3 cups fresh or frozen broccoli florets

¼ teaspoon ground nutmeg

½ teaspoon dry mustard

1 pinch cayenne pepper

4 cups low FODMAP vegetable broth (see Ingredient Tip)

1 cup shredded mild Cheddar cheese, aged 30 days or more

Sea salt and freshly ground black pepper to taste

Heat the avocado oil over medium heat in a saucepan large enough to hold all of the vegetables.

When the oil is shimmering but not smoking, add the green onions, celery, carrots, and 1½ cups of the broccoli. Sauté, stirring often, for 7 minutes or until the vegetables are beginning to soften.

Add the nutmeg, dry mustard, and cayenne and cook for 1 more minute. Add the vegetable broth, raise the heat to high, and bring to boil. Reduce the heat to a simmer and continue to cook for 10 minutes or until the vegetables are soft.

Using an immersion blender, blend the vegetables and broth until smooth.

Add the remaining 1½ cups of broccoli, raise the heat to medium-high, and bring the mixture to a boil. Reduce the heat to a simmer and cook for 7 more minutes or until the broccoli is tender.

Remove from the heat and stir in the Cheddar cheese until the cheese is melted fully and incorporated

Taste and then add salt and pepper.

**Ingredient Tip:**
I use Casa de Sante Vegetable Stock Powder to make a low FODMAP vegetable broth.

# Delicata Squash Soup

**Dairy-free, Gluten-free, Nut-free, Egg-free**

**Diets: BPD, CSD, LF, SCD, SSFG**

———

**Serves 4**

**Prep Time: 10 minutes/Cook Time: 60 minutes**

If you're having a hard time with your digestion, soup is often easier on the system because it's already a liquid. This soup includes coconut milk, a healthy fat that will keep you full longer.

2 delicata squash (about 1½ pounds total)

2 tablespoons avocado oil

4 green onions (green parts only), chopped

1 stalk celery, chopped

1 teaspoon ground coriander

1 teaspoon cumin

4 cups low FODMAP vegetable broth (see Ingredient Tip)

1 cup canned pumpkin

1 cup full-fat coconut milk (preferably without gums)

Freshly squeezed juice of 1 lime

4 teaspoons chopped fresh cilantro

Preheat the oven to 425°F. Line a rimmed baking sheet with parchment paper or aluminum foil.

Cut off the ends of the squash, cut them in half lengthwise, and remove the seeds.

Place the squash cut-sides down on the baking sheet and bake in the preheated oven for 35 minutes or until the flesh has softened.

When cool enough to handle, scoop out the flesh and set it aside.

Heat a medium saucepan over medium heat and add the avocado oil. Add the green onions and celery and cook for 5 minutes or until softened. Add the coriander and cumin and sauté for 1 more minute.

Add the broth, cooked squash, and pumpkin. Bring to boil, then reduce the heat to a simmer and cook for 10 minutes.

Remove from the heat and puree the soup with an immersion blender. Stir in the coconut milk and lime juice.

Ladle into bowls and top each bowl of soup with 1 teaspoon of cilantro.

### Ingredient Tip:

I use Casa de Sante Vegetable Stock Powder to make a low FODMAP vegetable broth.

### Variation:

You can substitute a different type of squash for the delicata if you wish. Some squash are more dense than others, so you can add more or less broth as needed. If you're one of those people who just hate cilantro, leave it off.

# Shivan's Soothing Soup

### Dairy-free, Gluten-free, Nut-free, Egg-free
### Diets: BPD, CSD, LF, SCD, SSFG

---

**Serves 2**
**Prep Time: 10 minutes/Cook Time: 30 minutes**

You can prep all the dry ingredients, bag them up, and freeze them until you're ready to cook your soup. Use organic ingredients whenever possible.

1 handful fresh spinach, washed and dried
1 whole butternut squash, peeled and diced
1 zucchini, diced
½ cup chopped leeks, green part only
Beet (1 thin slice)
1 sweet potato, peeled and diced
3 carrots, diced, with skin
1 vegetable bouillon cube without any garlic or onion (such as Casa de Sante)
2 quarts water

Prep the spinach, butternut squash, zucchini, leeks, beet, sweet potato, and carrots. Once prepped, put them in a quart-size freezer bag and freeze until you are ready to cook the soup.

Combine the bouillon cube and water in a pot large enough to hold all of the ingredients. Add the frozen vegetables and bring to a boil. Reduce the heat to a simmer and cook for 30 minutes or until the vegetables are soft.

Puree the soup or strain out the vegetables and drink the broth.

# Citrus and Roasted Fennel Salad

**Dairy-free, Gluten-free, Nut-free, Egg-free**

**Diets: BPD, CSD, LF, SCD, SSFG**

---

**Serves 4**

**Prep Time: 15 minutes/Cook Time: 15 minutes**

This salad is visually stunning, especially if you use citrus in a variety of colors. Along with navel oranges and tangerines, look for a small pink or yellow grapefruit and blood oranges, which will be a darker orange or red inside.

1 cup chopped fennel

1 tablespoon avocado oil

Sea salt and freshly ground black pepper to taste

2½ pounds of a variety of citrus, such as oranges, tangerines, or
   grapefruit

½ avocado, cubed

1 tablespoon chopped fresh chives

¼ cup extra-virgin olive oil

3 tablespoons champagne vinegar

1 tablespoon clover honey

1 tablespoon chopped mint leaves

Preheat the oven to 425°F. Line a rimmed baking sheet with parchment paper or aluminum foil.

Spread the fennel on the baking sheet, sprinkle with the avocado oil, and toss to coat it well.

Sprinkle the fennel lightly with salt and pepper and roast in the preheated oven for 15 minutes or until golden. Remove from the oven and set aside to cool.

Slice the peels off the citrus and then cut them crosswise into rounds. Place them on a serving platter and sprinkle the cooled fennel and avocado over the fruit.

In a small bowl, whisk the olive oil into the champagne vinegar until it is emulsified. Add the honey and whisk until incorporated.

Pour the dressing over the salad and top the salad with chopped mint leaves.

### SIBO Tip:

Eighty grams of grapefruit (approximately ⅓ cup) is considered low FODMAP on the latest version of the Monash University list even though it doesn't appear on the SSFG.

## Open-Faced Egg Salad Sandwich

**Dairy-free, Gluten-free, Nut-free**

**Diets: BPD, CSD, LF, SSFG\***

---

**Serves 4**

**Prep Time: 5 minutes/Cook Time: 30 minutes**

You can vary the salad by adding in any herbs you have on hand, such as tarragon, basil, cilantro, or parsley, and vegetables such as chopped cucumbers, green onions, cherry tomatoes, pickles, or bell peppers. If you don't tolerate rice cakes, put the salad in a lettuce cup or on SIBO-friendly crackers.

8 large eggs
⅓ cup SIBO-friendly mayonnaise
1 tablespoon SIBO-friendly mustard
1 teaspoon freshly squeezed lemon juice
½ stalk celery, finely chopped
2 tablespoons chopped fresh dill
2 tablespoons chopped fresh chives
½ teaspoon salt
¼ teaspoon freshly ground black pepper
4 SIBO-friendly rice cakes (no onion, garlic, or other high
    FODMAP ingredients)
Paprika for garnish

Place the eggs in a medium saucepan and cover them with cold water. Bring to a boil over medium heat and remove from the heat. Let the eggs stand in the hot water for 12 minutes.

Meanwhile, fill a medium bowl with cold water and ice cubes.

Transfer the eggs to the bowl of cold water until they are cool enough to handle. Peel and place the eggs in a medium bowl.

Mash the eggs with a fork and mix in the mayonnaise, mustard, lemon juice, celery, dill, chives, salt, and pepper.

Place one-quarter of the mixture on each rice cake and sprinkle with the paprika.

## Rainbow Veggie Spring Rolls with Almond Dipping Sauce

Dairy-free, Gluten-free, Egg-free

Diets: BPD, LF, SSFG*

---

**Serves 8**

Prep Time: 40 minutes

If you can't tolerate some of the herbs or vegetables in this roll, simply leave them out and add another ingredient that works better for you. If you want to eat one as a main meal, add some seared tofu for protein. If you're new to wrapping spring rolls, there are multiple online videos that demonstrate the process.

3 tablespoons sugar-free rice wine vinegar

2 tablespoons olive or avocado oil

⅓ cup almond butter or another nut butter of choice

2 tablespoons coconut aminos

1 tablespoon finely minced fresh ginger

8 round rice paper wrappers

4 leaves butter or red leaf lettuce, cleaned and torn in half

1 cup chopped fresh cilantro

24 fresh mint leaves

16 fresh basil leaves

2 small carrots, thinly sliced into matchstick pieces

1 cup red or purple cabbage, shredded fine

1 small English cucumber, peeled and thinly sliced into matchstick pieces

1 avocado, cut into thin slices

1 red bell pepper, thinly sliced into matchstick pieces

In a medium bowl, whisk together the rice wine vinegar, oil, nut butter, coconut aminos, and ginger and set aside.

Fill a rimmed baking sheet with warm water. Dip one rice paper wrapper in the water for a maximum of 5 seconds.

Set the rice paper on a cutting board or a baking sheet lined with parchment paper and place half of a lettuce leaf in the middle.

Spread one-eighth portion of the herbs and vegetables lengthwise down the middle of the lettuce.

Fold the short ends of the wrapper inward and gently roll the long edge as tightly as possible.

Set the roll aside and repeat for the remaining rolls.

Serve immediately with the dipping sauce.

**Ingredient Tip:**

Coconut aminos is a savory sauce that is available in many large markets as well as online.

**SIBO Tip:**

While white rice isn't on the SSFG, both white rice and white potato are on other SIBO diets and are often recommended for people who want to add more carbohydrates to their diet to avoid excessive weight loss. If you are going to try white rice or white rice products, start with a small amount and increase the portion size slowly to determine your tolerance.

# ENTRÉES

# Spaghetti Squash Lasagna

### Gluten-free, Nut-free, Egg-free

### Diets: BPD, CSD, LF, SCD, SSFG

---

### Serves 6

### Prep Time: 10 minutes/Cook Time: 1 hour and 40 minutes

This lasagna highlights low FODMAP spaghetti squash with all the familiar taste of traditional lasagna. It's great for a family dinner or to take to a potluck.

1 large spaghetti squash (about 4 pounds)

1 tablespoon avocado oil

2 cups SIBO-friendly canned tomato sauce (tomatoes only, such as Pomi)

2 tablespoons garlic oil (see page 124)

2 teaspoons Italian herbs (without garlic)

1 teaspoon dried fennel (optional)

1¼ teaspoons sea salt

½ teaspoon freshly ground black pepper

4 cups freshly grated white Cheddar cheese (aged at least 30 days)

1 cup freshly grated Parmesan cheese (aged at least 30 days)

Preheat the oven to 400°F. Line a baking sheet with parchment paper.

Cut the spaghetti squash in half widthwise. Remove the seeds and then cut each half in half. Brush each of the four pieces with ¾ teaspoon of the avocado oil.

Place the squash on the parchment paper cut-side down and use the tip of a sharp knife to poke several holes in each piece.

Roast the squash in the preheated oven for 60 minutes. Remove from the oven and set aside to cool. Reduce the oven temperature to 375°F. Using a fork, scrape the flesh off the squash rind and set it aside.

In a medium saucepan over medium heat, combine the tomato sauce, garlic oil, Italian herbs, fennel if desired, salt, and pepper. When the mixture is hot, reduce the heat to low and keep it warm.

In a medium mixing bowl, combine the Cheddar and Parmesan cheeses.

Spread 2 tablespoons of the sauce in the bottom of an 8 x 12-inch or 9 x 12-inch baking pan. This will prevent the squash from sticking to the pan.

Spread a third of the squash over the sauce. Add a third of the remaining sauce and a third of the cheese. Repeat twice, ending with a layer of cheese.

Bake for 40 minutes or until the cheese is golden brown on top.

Allow the lasagna to rest for 10 minutes before cutting.

# Mexican Baked Potato

Gluten-free, Nut-free, Egg-free

Diets: CSD, LF, SSFG*

———

**Serves 2**

Prep Time: 10 minutes/Cook Time: 1 hour and 15 minutes

Potatoes aren't listed on the SSFG, but Dr. Siebecker typically recommends white rice or peeled white potatoes for those who tolerate starch and want more carbohydrates in their diet. According to Monash University, white potatoes are low FODMAPs (however, the skins contain fiber, which is fermentable).

2 small russet potatoes, washed and dried

2 teaspoons avocado oil

1 teaspoon sea salt

1 tablespoon olive oil

1 small red bell pepper, seeded and chopped

1 small zucchini, peeled (if desired), halved lengthwise, and
 chopped

½ teaspoon ground cumin

1 tablespoon salted butter

2 tablespoons 24-Hour Yogurt (page 138), plus more for topping

¼ cup freshly grated Cheddar cheese (aged 30 days or more)

1 tablespoon chopped fresh cilantro

2 green onions (green parts only), chopped

2 tablespoons SIBO-friendly salsa or chopped tomatoes

Preheat the oven to 350°F. Line a baking sheet with aluminum foil.

Prick each potato with a fork in eight different places. Coat each potato with 1 teaspoon of avocado oil and rub each with ¼ teaspoon salt.

Place the potatoes directly on the middle oven rack and the baking sheet on the rack below.

Cook the potatoes for 1 hour or until the skin is crisp and the flesh is easily pierced with a knife.

Transfer the cooked potatoes to two dinner plates.

Heat the olive oil in a medium sauté pan over medium-high heat. Add the bell pepper and cook, stirring often, for 4 minutes or until it begins to soften. Add the zucchini, cumin, and ½ teaspoon of the remaining salt and cook another 3 to 5 minutes, stirring frequently. Remove from the heat and set aside.

Cut each potato almost from end to end, without fully cutting them in half. Squeeze the ends toward each other to loosen the flesh from the skin. Fluff the flesh with a fork.

Place 1½ teaspoons butter, 1 tablespoon yogurt, and 1 tablespoon cheese in each potato. Mix the toppings into the potato flesh.

Top the potatoes with the vegetable mixture, cilantro, green onion, salsa, and the remaining cheese.

# Buddha Bowl

**Gluten-free, Nut-free**

**Diets: BPD, CSD, LF, SSFG\***

---

**Serves 4**

**Prep Time: 10 minutes/Cook Time: 25 minutes**

You can substitute different vegetables in this recipe depending on what you tolerate best. Or, if you are not digesting raw vegetables well, use mostly cooked vegetables and few or no raw items. It's important to eat as many foods as possible on any SIBO diet to support your microbiome, so even having small amounts of a variety of vegetables is important.

3 cups broccoli florets

3 cups sliced carrots

2 tablespoons olive oil

Sea salt to taste

4 cups warm cooked White Rice (page 179) or Easy Pesto Rice (page 180)

1 small English cucumber, peeled and sliced thin

4 large hard-boiled eggs, halved

1 cup chopped red cabbage

1 cup chopped fresh spinach

2 tablespoons fresh microgreens

2 tablespoons chopped fresh chives

1 tablespoon chopped fresh flat-leaf parsley

Green Goddess Dressing (page 204)

½ avocado, peeled and sliced

Preheat the oven to 400°F. Line a rimmed baking sheet with parchment paper or aluminum foil.

Spread the broccoli and carrots on the baking sheet. Toss with the olive oil and sprinkle with the salt.

Bake for 10 minutes. Flip the vegetables as best as you can and bake for 10 more minutes. Remove from the oven and set aside to cool.

Meanwhile, place 1 cup of warm rice in each of four bowls. Spoon the cooked vegetables over the rice.

Divide the cucumber, egg halves, cabbage, and spinach equally among the four bowls, arranging the items in separate sections. Top each bowl with equal amounts of the microgreens, chives, and Green Goddess Dressing.

Top with the avocado slices and serve.

**Ingredient Tip:**
While most of the ingredients in this recipe are dairy-free, there is dairy in the yogurt used in the Green Goddess Dressing recipe. If you prefer a dairy-free version, leave out the yogurt and choose another dressing, such as the almond sauce in the Rainbow Veggie Spring Rolls (page 165).

# Cheesy Veggie Frittata

Dairy-free, Gluten-free, Nut-free

Diets: BPD, LF, SCD, SSFG

---

### Serves 6 to 8

Prep Time: 15 minutes/Cook Time: 50 minutes

I've listed the frittata in the entrée section because I believe it would be wrong to relegate it to breakfast alone!

1 red bell pepper, diced

1 yellow bell pepper, diced

1 cup chopped broccoli florets

2 tablespoons garlic oil (see page 124)

1 tablespoon avocado oil

2 teaspoons sea salt

½ teaspoon freshly ground black pepper

12 large eggs

¾ cup SIBO-friendly milk

½ cup freshly grated Parmesan cheese (optional)

2 tablespoons (¼ stick) salted butter or coconut oil

¼ cup chopped green onions (green parts only)

1 cup finely chopped spinach

½ cup shredded carrots

1 cup Gruyère cheese (optional)

Preheat the oven to 400°F. Line a rimmed baking sheet with parchment paper or aluminum foil.

Spread the bell peppers and the broccoli on the baking sheet and sprinkle with the garlic oil and avocado oil. Toss to coat the vegetables and then sprinkle with 1 teaspoon of the salt and the black pepper.

Bake for 15 minutes. Remove from the oven and set aside. Reduce the oven heat to 350°F.

In a large bowl, whisk together the eggs, milk, 1 remaining teaspoon of salt, and the Parmesan cheese if desired.

Melt the butter in a 10-inch ovenproof skillet (a cast-iron skillet works well) over medium heat.

When the butter is melted, add the green onions, spinach, and carrots and sauté for 2 minutes.

Add the reserved broccoli and bell peppers and toss the vegetables until well combined.

Reduce the heat to low, pour the egg mixture over the vegetables, and cook for 2 minutes without stirring.

Transfer the pan to the oven and bake for 25 minutes or until the frittata is set in the middle.

Sprinkle the frittata with the Gruyère if using and bake for another 3 minutes or until the cheese is melted and starting to bubble.

Remove from the oven, cut into six or eight wedges, and serve immediately.

**Cooking Tip:**

A frittata is an excellent way to use any leftover roasted vegetables you have on hand. Harder vegetables should always be roasted first, while softer vegetables such as spinach can be sautéed in a pan before adding the eggs.

# Shepherd's Pie

### Dairy-free, Gluten-free, Nut-free, Egg-free

### Diets: BPD, LF, SSFG*

---

### Serves 6

### Prep Time: 15 minutes/Cook Time: 50 minutes

Shepherd's pie is comfort food at its best and a great way to use up extra mashed potatoes. (See notes about potato in Mexican Baked Potato [page 170].) I've added lentils to this version, giving it some extra protein and extra taste.

2 pounds Yukon Gold potatoes, peeled and halved

6 tablespoons (¾ stick) unsalted butter, ghee, or coconut oil (or use Herb Compound Butter [page 205])

½ cup SIBO-friendly milk

½ teaspoon sea salt, or more as needed

2 tablespoons garlic oil (see page 124)

1 stalk celery, chopped

2 carrots, chopped

1 red bell pepper, seeded and chopped

1 cup finely chopped spinach

6 green onions (green parts only), chopped

1 tablespoon tomato paste

1 teaspoon dried thyme

½ teaspoon smoked paprika

¾ cup low FODMAP vegetable broth (see Ingredient Tip)

One 15-ounce can lentils, rinsed and drained

½ teaspoon freshly ground black pepper

Place the potatoes in a medium or large saucepan and add enough water to cover the potatoes.

Bring to a boil over high heat, then reduce the heat to medium-high and cook for 20 minutes or until the potatoes are soft and easily pierced with a fork.

Drain the potatoes and transfer them to a large bowl. Add the butter, milk, and salt.

Using a handheld mixer with the whisk attachment, blend the potatoes, butter, milk, and salt until almost smooth. Taste and add more salt as needed. Set aside.

Preheat the oven to 400°F.

Heat the garlic oil in a large sauté pan over medium-high heat for 1 minute. Add the celery, carrots, and bell pepper to the pan and sauté for 7 minutes or until they begin to soften. Add the spinach and green onions and sauté 1 more minute. Add the tomato paste, thyme, and paprika and sauté for another minute. Add the vegetable broth and lentils. Add the black pepper.

Mix to combine all of the ingredients, remove from the heat, taste, and add more salt if needed.

Transfer the vegetable mixture to a pie pan or an 8-inch-square baking pan.

Cover the vegetables evenly with the mashed potatoes and bake the pie in the preheated oven for 20 minutes.

**Ingredient Tip:**

I use Casa de Sante Vegetable Stock Powder to make a low FODMAP vegetable broth.

**SIBO Tip:**

We use canned and drained lentils in this recipe because, according to Monash University, when foods are canned, the FODMAPs leach out into the canning water.

# SIDE DISHES

# White Rice

Dairy-free, Gluten-free, Nut-free, Egg-free
Diets: BPD, CSD, LF, SSFG*

---

**Serves 4**

Prep Time: 5 minutes/Cook Time: 20 minutes

You can always use water to cook your rice, but try broth for added taste and nutrient density or coconut milk for added taste and healthy fat. Although these instructions work for most types of medium-grain rice, double-check the package instructions to see if the manufacturer recommends a different cooking time.

2 cups water, broth, or coconut milk
1 teaspoon sea salt (unless using salted broth)
1 cup medium-grain white rice (such as jasmine or basmati)
2 tablespoons ghee, butter, coconut oil, olive oil, or Herb
    Compound Butter (page 205)

Pour the water and salt into a medium pan with a lid and bring to a boil over high heat.

Add the rice and stir. Reduce the heat to medium-low, cover, and cook for 20 minutes without stirring or uncovering.

Remove the pan from the heat, fluff the rice with a fork, drain off any excess liquid, and stir in the ghee.

# Easy Pesto Rice

### Dairy-free, Gluten-free, Nut-free, Egg-free

### Diets: BPD, CSD, LF, SSFG*

---

### Serves 4

### Prep Time: 5 minutes/Cook Time: 5 minutes

This recipe will make more than enough pesto, so you can use the rest as a dip, over roasted vegetables, or on zucchini noodles. It will keep, tightly covered, in the refrigerator for up to 1 week.

¼ cup garlic oil (see page 124)

¼ cup olive oil

1 tablespoon freshly squeezed lemon juice

6 ounces fresh organic basil or spinach, washed and dried

1 teaspoon sea salt

¼ teaspoon freshly cracked black pepper (optional)

¼ cup walnuts or pine nuts (optional)

¼ cup freshly grated Parmesan cheese (optional)

2 cups cooked brown or white rice

Place the garlic oil, olive oil, lemon juice, basil, salt, pepper, walnuts, and Parmesan in the bowl of a food processor.

Process until fairly smooth, scraping down the sides of the container as necessary.

Combine the warm rice with ½ cup of the pesto and serve immediately.

### Ingredient Tip:

Basil is harder to find in the winter, so using spinach instead makes pesto an option all year round.

# Pineapple Fried Rice

Dairy-free, Gluten-free, Nut-free, Egg-free

Diets: BPD, CSD, LF, SSFG*

---

**Serves 4**

Prep Time: 10 minutes/Cook Time: 20 minutes

It can be particularly challenging when you aren't able to enjoy favorite comfort foods like fried rice. In this recipe, we've removed the gluten and soy but maintained the delicious flavor.

1 large egg yolk

2 cups cooked and cooled white rice

1 tablespoon plus 1 teaspoon coconut oil

2 large whole eggs

1½ cups diced fresh pineapple

1 medium organic bell pepper, seeded and diced

¾ cup chopped green onions (green parts only)

½ cup roasted slivered almonds

2 tablespoons coconut aminos (see Ingredient Tip, page 166)

1 teaspoon SIBO-friendly hot sauce, such as McIlhenny Tabasco (optional)

1 teaspoon garlic oil (see page 124)

In a medium mixing bowl, mix the egg yolk into the cooled white rice so that all of the rice is coated. Set aside.

In a large sauté pan or skillet, heat 1 teaspoon of the coconut oil over medium heat.

Crack the 2 whole eggs into a small bowl and whisk.

Add the eggs to the pan with the coconut oil and stir for 4 to 5 minutes, until cooked. Remove the scrambled eggs from the pan and set aside.

Place the remaining 1 tablespoon of coconut oil in the same pan and set over medium heat.

Add the pineapple and bell pepper and sauté for 3 to 5 minutes, until the bell pepper begins to soften. Add the green onions and sauté for another minute. Add the egg yolk–coated rice, almonds, coconut aminos, and hot sauce, if using, and cook, stirring, for 5 minutes or until the egg is cooked.

Return the scrambled eggs to the pan along with the garlic oil and stir to combine.

**SIBO Tip:**

Even though the SSFG doesn't include rice, Dr. Siebecker herself recommends white rice to those who tolerate grains in their diet and for those trying to avoid weight loss. White rice is high glycemic, which means that it is metabolized quickly and is therefore a low-fermentable food. Store leftovers in the freezer to prevent the rice from becoming gummy.

# Crispy Accordion Potatoes

Gluten-free, Nut-free, Egg-free

Diets: BPD, CSD, LF, SSFG*

---

**Serves 4**

Prep Time: 15 minutes/Cook Time: 1 hour and 15 minutes

You can also top these potatoes with additional ingredients such as 24-Hour Yogurt (page 138), chimichurri sauce, or hollandaise sauce.

4 Yukon Gold or small russet potatoes (about 1½ pounds total)
2 tablespoons garlic oil (see page 124)
Sea salt and freshly ground black pepper to taste
2 tablespoons (¼ stick) salted butter
1 tablespoon chopped flat-leaf parsley

Preheat the oven to 425°F. Line a baking sheet with aluminum foil or parchment paper and set aside.

Slice the potatoes three-quarters of the way through at ⅛-inch intervals.

Place the potatoes on the baking sheet and brush between the slices with the garlic oil. Sprinkle with salt and black pepper. Bake for 1 hour and 15 minutes or until golden and cooked through.

While the potatoes are baking, melt the butter in a small pan and set aside.

Transfer the cooked potatoes to a serving plate, drizzle with the melted butter, and sprinkle with the parsley.

**SIBO Tip:**
Peeling the potatoes in this recipe is optional, but if you have just started on a SIBO diet or you know you don't do well with fiber, it's recommended that you peel them so that they're easier to digest.

# Easy Mashed Potatoes

### Dairy-free, Gluten-free, Nut-free, Egg-free

### Diets: BPD, CSD, LF, SSFG*

---

### Serves 4

#### Prep Time: 5 minutes/Cook Time: 25 minutes

Including potatoes in a SIBO diet is a great way to add high-glycemic carbohydrates that are not so likely to ferment and feed bacteria. However, not everyone reacts well to the starch in potatoes, so start with a small amount to assess your tolerance.

2 pounds Yukon Gold potatoes
½ cup ghee or salted or unsalted butter at room temperature, olive oil, or coconut oil
⅔ cup broth or SIBO-friendly milk of your choice, warmed
1 teaspoon sea salt, or more as needed

Peel the potatoes and place them in a large pot. Add enough water to fully cover the potatoes and set over high heat. Bring to a boil and then reduce the heat to medium-high.

Cook the potatoes for 20 minutes or until they are fork-tender but not falling apart.

Drain and transfer the potatoes to a medium bowl. Add the ghee, broth, and salt and whisk with a handheld electric mixer until smooth. Taste and add additional salt if desired.

**Ingredient Tip:**
To make garlic mashed potatoes, substitute 2 tablespoons garlic oil (see page 124) for the ghee in this recipe.

# Roasted Delicata Squash
# with Five Spice Powder

**Dairy-free, Gluten-free, Nut-free, Egg Free**

**Diets: BPD, CSD, LF, SCD, SSFG**

---

**Serves 4**

**Prep Time: 5 minutes/Cook Time: 25 minutes**

You don't have to peel a delicata squash, as the peel is edible and softens when cooked. But if you are just starting a SIBO diet, you can peel it just so it will be easier for you to digest.

1 large or two small delicata squash (1 pound total)

2 tablespoons olive oil

1 teaspoon five spice powder

1 teaspoon sea salt

½ teaspoon freshly ground black pepper

Preheat the oven to 425°F. Line a rimmed baking sheet with parchment paper.

Scrub the squash (assuming you're not peeling it), cut off the ends, cut the squash in half lengthwise, and remove the seeds. Cut each half squash into ½-inch-thick slices.

Transfer the slices to the baking sheet and sprinkle with the olive oil, five spice powder, salt, and pepper and toss to coat it evenly.

Bake for 15 minutes, then turn over the slices and return to the oven for 10 more minutes or until cooked through and soft.

## SIBO Tip:

At this time, delicata squash has not been tested by Monash University, so the particular low FODMAP amounts are unknown. However, as with all foods, it's best to start with small amounts and increase them as tolerated.

## Pureed Carrots

Dairy-free, Gluten-free, Nut-free, Egg-free

Diets: BPD, CSD, LF, SCD, SSFG

---

**Serves 4**

Prep Time: 5 minutes/Cook Time: 25 minutes

This recipe can be adapted to suit your preferences. Add some cinnamon and clover honey for a delicious breakfast dish. Add a spice such as cumin or some grated fresh ginger to give it a different flavor profile.

4 cups peeled and chopped carrots
3 tablespoons coconut oil or olive oil
¼ teaspoon sea salt, or more as needed
Freshly ground black pepper to taste

Steam the carrots for 20 minutes or until they are soft but not mushy.

Transfer the carrots to the bowl of a food processor, add the coconut oil, salt, and pepper, and blend until smooth.

Taste and add more salt, pepper, or other spices if desired.

# Cheesy Baked Carrot Fries with Ranch Dressing

Gluten-free, Nut-free, Egg-free

Diets: BPD, LF, SCD, SSFG

---

**Serves 4**

Prep Time: 15 minutes/Cook Time: 20 minutes

These cheesy carrot fries will hit the spot when you need a salty, cheesy but SIBO-friendly side dish. You won't need the entire amount of Ranch Dressing, but it can also be used for side salads or as a dip for other roasted vegetables. It will keep in the refrigerator for up to 1 week.

### For the Ranch Dressing:

1 cup 24-Hour Yogurt (page 138)

1 tablespoon garlic oil (see page 124)

1 tablespoon chopped fresh chives or 1 teaspoon dried

1 tablespoon chopped fresh flat-leaf parsley or 1 teaspoon dried

1 tablespoon chopped fresh dill or 1 teaspoon dried

¼ cup freshly grated Parmesan cheese (optional)

¼ teaspoon sea salt, or more as needed

Freshly ground black pepper to taste

### For the Carrot Fries:

4 carrots, peeled and cut into sticks (like French fries)

1 tablespoon garlic oil (see page 124)

½ cup plus 1 tablespoon freshly grated Parmesan cheese

1 teaspoon sea salt

½ teaspoon freshly ground black pepper

¼ cup chopped fresh flat-leaf parsley

Make the dressing: Combine the yogurt, garlic oil, chives, parsley, dill, cheese if using, salt, and pepper in a small bowl. Taste and add more salt if needed. Set aside. The ranch dressing can be made up to a day in advance.

Make the carrots: Preheat the oven to 425°F. Line a rimmed baking sheet with parchment paper.

Place the carrot sticks on the baking sheet and top with the garlic oil, ½ cup of the Parmesan, salt, and pepper. Toss to evenly coat the carrots. Bake for 20 minutes.

Transfer to a serving plate. Sprinkle with the remaining 1 tablespoon of Parmesan and the chopped parsley.

Serve with the ranch dip.

# DESSERTS

# Honey Macaroons

**Dairy-free, Gluten-free, Nut-free**

**Diets: BPD, CSD, LF, SCD, SSFG**

---

**Makes 30 cookies**

**Prep Time: 10 minutes/Cook Time: 30 minutes**

If you've ever wondered about the difference between macaroons and macarons, it's that macaroons are made with coconut and macarons are made with almond flour.

5 large egg whites

¼ teaspoon sea salt

½ cup clover honey

1 tablespoon vanilla extract

3 cups shredded unsweetened coconut

Zest of 1 organic lemon

1 cup dairy-free chocolate chips (optional)

2 teaspoons olive oil

Preheat the oven to 350°F. Line two baking sheets with parchment paper.

Place the egg whites and salt in a large mixing bowl and beat with an electric mixer for 5 minutes, until they are shiny and form stiff peaks. Stir in the honey, vanilla, coconut, and lemon zest until incorporated.

Scoop tablespoon-size rounds of mixture and place them on the prepared baking sheets.

Bake in the preheated oven for 15 minutes, or until the macaroons are lightly browned at the peaks and on the bottom. Transfer the baking sheets to cooling racks and cool the cookies completely.

Melt the chocolate chips, if desired, in a small saucepan over low heat, stirring often. Using a teaspoon, drizzle each macaroon with a bit of melted chocolate. Refrigerate for 10 minutes until the chocolate is firm.

The macaroons will keep in an airtight container at room temperature for up to 4 days.

**SIBO Tips:**

Coconut can be hard for some people to digest. If you're unsure of your tolerance, start with just one cookie to see how your system reacts. You may wind up having to give the rest of the batch to a friend or coworker, but, when you have SIBO, that's the way the cookie sometimes crumbles. Or you could freeze them and try one again after about a month. Just because you don't tolerate a particular food on the first try doesn't mean you won't be okay with it as you heal.

If you're following the SCD diet, do not use the chocolate chips.

## Zesty Lime Pie

### Dairy-free, Gluten-free

### Diets: BPD, CSD, SCD, SSFG

---

### Serves 8

### Prep Time: 10 minutes/Cook Time: 35 minutes

If you prefer a lemon curd, you can easily substitute lemon juice and zest for the lime juice and zest. This pie can be topped with fruit compote, such as blueberry, or a SIBO-friendly whipped topping.

¼ cup melted ghee, salted or unsalted butter, or coconut oil, cooled
  to room temperature, plus ¾ cup ghee, butter, or coconut milk
1½ cups almond flour, packed
½ teaspoon sea salt
1 teaspoon ground cinnamon
⅔ cup plus 2 tablespoons clover honey
6 large eggs
2 tablespoons lime zest
1 cup freshly squeezed lime juice

Place a fine mesh sieve over a medium bowl and set aside. Preheat the oven to 350°F.

Combine ¼ cup of the melted ghee, almond flour, salt, cinnamon, and 2 tablespoons of the honey in a medium bowl and mix thoroughly.

Transfer the mixture to a pie plate and, with your fingers, press it down and toward the edges to form a crust. Bake the crust for 15 minutes. Remove from the oven and set aside.

In a medium saucepan, whisk together the remaining ⅔ cup honey, the eggs, and lime zest.

Add the lime juice and mix to incorporate.

Set the saucepan on the stove over medium heat. Add the remaining ¾ cup ghee and whisk it into the mixture while it melts. Stir the mixture until it is thick enough to coat the back of a spoon and bubbles rise to the surface.

Remove from the heat and pour the curd through the sieve into the bowl. Once all of the curd is in the bowl, pour it into the prepared piecrust.

Refrigerate for several hours before serving.

**SIBO Tip:**

This recipe isn't considered low FODMAP because of the amount of honey it includes, but many people with SIBO tolerate honey quite well. Before you bake this pie, try honey by itself to see if you tolerate it.

# Orange Cinnamon Rice Pudding

Dairy-free, Gluten-free, Nut-free, Egg-free

Diets: BPD, CSD, LF, SSFG*

---

**Serves 8**

Prep Time: 5 minutes/Cook Time: 25 minutes

This rice pudding is creamy and comforting. It makes a delicious dessert but is also great as a snack, or for breakfast with some protein on the side.

3 cups SIBO-friendly milk

1 cup full-fat coconut milk

1 cup short- or medium-grain white rice

Zest of 1 organic orange

1 teaspoon ground cinnamon

½ teaspoon ground nutmeg

½ teaspoon sea salt

3 tablespoons clover honey (or maple syrup if not following the SSFG)

1 teaspoon vanilla extract

Place SIBO-friendly milk, coconut milk, rice, orange zest, cinnamon, nutmeg, and salt in a medium saucepan over medium-high heat. Bring to a boil and then reduce the heat to a simmer.

Simmer, stirring occasionally, for 20 minutes or until the rice is cooked and the mixture thickens into a pudding. Stir more frequently as the liquid evaporates to make sure the rice doesn't stick to the bottom of the pan.

Remove from the heat and add the honey and vanilla.

Cool and serve warm or chilled. The pudding will keep, tightly covered, in the refrigerator for up to 1 week.

**Ingredient Tip:**
This pudding has a light sweetness, but you can add more or less honey depending on your tolerance and taste preference.

# Ginger Almond Cookies

**Dairy-free, Gluten-free**

**Diets: BPD, CSD, LF, SCD, SSFG**

---

**Makes 2 dozen cookies**

Prep Time: 10 minutes/Cook Time: 14 minutes

These chewy cookies have a nice gingery taste without being overpowering. Since they are relatively flat, they pack or freeze well.

½ teaspoon baking soda

¼ teaspoon sea salt

2 tablespoons coconut flour

1 teaspoon ground ginger

1 cup almond butter

½ cup clover honey

1 large egg, lightly beaten

1 tablespoon finely chopped fresh ginger

Sea salt flakes (optional)

Preheat the oven to 350°F.

Line two baking sheets with parchment paper.

Combine the baking soda, salt, and coconut flour in a medium bowl and stir until well mixed. Add the almond butter, honey, egg, and ginger and mix well.

Scoop 12 heaping teaspoonfuls of dough, spaced evenly apart, onto each baking sheet.

Sprinkle the cookies with salt flakes if desired and bake in the preheated oven for 12 to 14 minutes, until the cookies are golden.

Transfer the baking sheets to cooling racks and allow the cookies to cool on the baking sheets.

**Ingredient Tips:**

If you tolerate chocolate chips, you can add ½ cup to the dough if desired.

Sea salt flakes are larger (flakier) than regular sea salt and have a nice mouthfeel on cookies, but you can use regular sea salt as well.

# Chocolate-Covered Bananas

### Dairy-free, Gluten-free, Nut-free, Egg-free

### Diets: CSD, LF, SSFG*

---

### Serves 4

#### Prep Time: 10 minutes/Cook Time: 10 minutes

You can either refrigerate or freeze these bananas—some people prefer the texture of a frozen banana while others enjoy them less solid. The SSFG doesn't specifically include chocolate, but many people with SIBO do well with small amounts of dark chocolate. If you are not sure of your tolerance level, start with a small amount.

### Special Equipment:

4 POPSICLE STICKS OR CHOPSTICKS

2 ripe but still firm bananas

1 cup dark dairy-free chocolate chips

2 teaspoons avocado olive or walnut oil

Optional toppings: Grain-Free Granola (page 142), chopped nuts, coconut flakes, shredded coconut, or mini dairy-free chocolate chips

Line a baking sheet with parchment paper.

Cut the bananas in half crosswise and insert a Popsicle stick or chopstick into the cut end of each half. Place the banana halves on the baking sheet and refrigerate or freeze for 15 minutes.

In a double boiler or a small saucepan set over low heat, melt the chocolate chips with the avocado oil, stirring frequently.

Place the optional toppings of your choice on separate plates.

Spoon the chocolate over each frozen banana half and immediately roll them in the topping of choice.

Return the bananas to the baking sheet and freeze for 30 minutes or until the chocolate sets.

Serve immediately, store in the refrigerator for up to 2 days, or freeze for up to 1 week.

### SIBO Diet Tip:

Depending on the diet you follow, a banana in a specific stage of ripeness may or may not be recommended. On the SSFG, bananas are listed as "fresh," meaning a banana in any stage of ripening. However, on SCD, only ripe bananas with brown spots are acceptable. According to the Monash low FODMAP app, one medium unripe banana is low FODMAP while no more than one-third of a medium ripe banana is low FODMAP. Confusing, right? The best thing to do is to try small amounts of ripe or unripe bananas and see what you can tolerate. I've had the best luck with bananas that are all yellow, without brown or green.

# SAUCES AND CONDIMENTS

Sauces and condiments are the false eyelashes of food—small changes that make a big impact. I have never appreciated mustard as much as I do in this phase of my dietary life.

# Quick and Easy Aioli

Dairy-free, Gluten-free, Nut-free

Diets: BPD, CSD, LF, SCD, SSFG

---

**Makes 1¼ cups**

**Prep Time: 7 minutes**

Aioli is a delicious lemony, garlicky mayonnaise that tastes better than you ever thought mayonnaise could. This recipe is SIBO-friendly, since it calls for garlic oil and not raw garlic. You can serve it as is or add an herb, such as dill, for an additional kick. It's delicious on raw or cooked vegetables, and you can use it as a dip for just about anything you could think of. It will keep, tightly covered, in the refrigerator for up to 3 days.

1 large pasteurized egg

½ teaspoon SIBO-friendly mustard

Freshly squeezed juice of 1 lemon

½ teaspoon sea salt

½ cup garlic oil (see page 124)

½ cup avocado oil

Combine the egg, mustard, lemon juice, and salt in the bowl of a food processor and mix at high speed for 2 minutes.

Pour the garlic oil and avocado oil through the food pusher in the top portion of the food processor. There is a small hole in the pusher that will allow the oil to drip through slowly.

Continue to mix as the oil drips in. Once all of the oil has been added, stop the processor and transfer the aioli to a small bowl. Use at once or store in the refrigerator for up to 2 days.

**Note:**

I like to use pasteurized eggs because it reduces the risk of salmonella—and remember, we all should be avoiding food poisoning!

# Thousand Island Dressing

Dairy-free, Gluten-free, Nut-free, Egg-free

Diets: BPD, CSD, LF, SCD, SSFG

---

**Makes ½ cup**

Prep Time: 5 minutes

Thousand island dressing isn't just for salad. It's also delicious on baked potatoes, on grilled cheese sandwiches, with crackers, or with vegetables.

½ cup SIBO-friendly mayonnaise

2 tablespoons SIBO-friendly ketchup

1 tablespoon apple cider vinegar

2 teaspoons clover honey

⅛ teaspoon sea salt

Freshly ground black pepper to taste

2 tablespoons SIBO-friendly relish

1 tablespoon finely chopped fresh chives

In a small bowl, whisk together the mayonnaise, ketchup, vinegar, honey, salt, and pepper. Stir in the relish and chives until incorporated. Serve immediately or store in the refrigerator for up to 1 week.

# Green Goddess Dressing

Dairy-free, Gluten-free, Nut-free, Egg-free

Diets: BPD, CSD, LF, SCD, SSFG

---

**Makes 1¼ cups**

**Prep Time: 10 minutes**

This dressing is said to have originated at the Palace Hotel in San Francisco, when the chef wanted to pay tribute to the actor George Arliss, who was then starring in a play titled *The Green Goddess.* Both the play and the dressing were hits then, and at least the dressing is still a hit today.

1 cup fresh flat-leaf parsley leaves
1 packed cup fresh spinach leaves
2 tablespoons tarragon leaves
3 tablespoons minced fresh chives
3 tablespoons freshly squeezed lemon juice
1 tablespoon champagne vinegar
¼ cup garlic oil (see page 124)
¼ cup avocado oil
¼ cup SIBO-friendly mayonnaise
¼ cup 24-Hour Yogurt (page 138)
½ teaspoon sea salt
Freshly ground black pepper to taste

Combine the parsley, spinach, tarragon, chives, lemon juice, vinegar, garlic oil, avocado oil, mayonnaise, yogurt, salt, and pepper in a blender and blend until smooth.

Serve immediately or keep tightly covered in the refrigerator for up to 3 days.

# Herb Compound Butter

Gluten-free, Nut-free, Egg-free

Diets: BPD, CSD, LF, SCD, SSFG

---

**Makes ½ cup**

Prep Time: 10 minutes

Herb butter is delicious on grilled, roasted, or steamed vegetables. It keeps well in the refrigerator or freezer and you can easily cut off a few pieces at a time. I used to think this type of "fancy" butter was just for holidays, but if you have SIBO, you have to pull out all the stops to make eating enjoyable. The sweet version is also amazingly satisfying.

½ cup (1 stick) salted butter, at room temperature
1 teaspoon chopped fresh rosemary
2 teaspoons chopped fresh chives
2 teaspoons chopped fresh flat-leaf parsley
1 teaspoon chopped fresh thyme

Place the butter, rosemary, chives, parsley, and thyme in a medium bowl and mix thoroughly with a spoon.

Use a spatula to remove the butter mixture from the bowl and place it on a piece of wax paper.

Form it into a log and wrap the paper around it. Refrigerate or freeze until needed.

## Ingredient Tip:

Try making a sweet version of this butter with clover honey or maple syrup and orange rind instead of the herbs. If you don't tolerate dairy well, you can always use coconut oil instead of the butter.

# Tapenade

Dairy-free, Gluten-free, Nut-free, Egg-free

Diets: BPD, CSD, LF, SCD, SSFG

---

**Makes ¾ cup**

Prep Time: 10 minutes

Tapenade makes a great dip for SIBO-friendly crackers or vegetables. It's delicious over grilled vegetables or a protein of your choice.

2 tablespoons garlic oil (see page 124)

One 12-ounce jar kalamata olives

2 tablespoons drained capers

¼ teaspoon dried Italian herbs without garlic

Place the garlic oil, olives, capers, and herbs in the bowl of a food processor and blend until pureed but still slightly chunky.

Scrape the tapenade from the processor with a spatula and serve it immediately or store tightly covered in the refrigerator for up to 1 week.

## SIBO Tip:

When looking for jarred items such as olives, capers, or spices, make sure there aren't added ingredients, such as garlic, that many people don't tolerate well.

# Lavender Simple Syrup

Dairy-free, Gluten-free, Nut-free, Egg-free

Diets: BPD—Phase I, CSD, LF, SCD, SSFG

---

**Makes I cup**

Prep Time: 5 minutes/Cook Time: 40 minutes

This simple syrup can also be made without the lavender or you can use other herbs, such as thyme or basil, and use it to flavor lemonade. If you want to be really lazy, you can buy it online, but it's extremely easy to make. Culinary lavender is available at organic grocery stores, at Whole Foods, and online.

½ cup clover honey
1 tablespoon culinary lavender, organic if possible

In a small saucepan, combine ½ cup water with the honey and lavender and set it over medium heat. Stir frequently until the honey is liquefied and mixed with the water.

Remove from the heat and let stand for 30 minutes. Strain the mixture through a fine mesh sieve to remove the bits of lavender.

Use the strained syrup at once or store it, tightly covered, in the refrigerator for up to 1 week.

**Cooking Tip:**
You can make larger batches so long as you maintain a fifty-fifty ratio of honey to water.

# AFTERWORD

I no longer *suffer* from SIBO. With the help of wonderful, dedicated doctors and nutritionists, I've learned how to manage my condition, and when symptoms flare up—as they will—I know what to do to overcome them.

My goal is that this book will help you to do the same. If you have symptoms of IBS but have never heard of SIBO, you'll now know for the first time what's been causing your symptoms. If you've just learned that you have SIBO, you won't have to repeat all the missteps I took or go down the wrong roads I traveled, because I've already identified them for you. If you've known for some time that you have it and haven't gotten the help you needed, I hope this book can be that help.

My purpose is to empower you to take control of your own health, and, if necessary, take this book to your doctor so that he or she can learn more about how to help you. Be sure to visit my website, sibosos .com, for more resources and information. The SOS stands for Save Our Selves. Each time we pick up a book, search online, and most importantly, take action, we're doing just that: saving our selves.

If you hear yourself saying the words "I've tried everything," ask yourself this: "Have I really, really tried everything?" There is always another stone to overturn and another place to look. You have a mission to accomplish in this world; don't let your health hold you back from achieving that. Don't give up. You deserve to be well.

*xoxo, Shivan*

# APPENDIX

## The SIBO Specific Food Guide for Vegetarians

*Adapted from Dr. Allison Siebecker's SIBO Specific Food Guide*

## VEGETABLES

LESS FERMENTABLE ➤ MORE FERMENTABLE

| "Green Foods"— SCD Legal, LOW FODMAP | "Yellow Foods"— SCD Legal, MODERATE FODMAP | "Orange Foods"—SCD Legal, HIGH FODMAP | "Red Foods"—SCD Illegal, HIGH FODMAP |
|---|---|---|---|
| Artichoke hearts*, ⅛ cup | Artichoke hearts*, ¼ cup | Artichoke | Bean sprouts |
| Arugula | Asparagus, 1 spear | Asparagus, 4 spears | Canned vegetables |
| Bamboo shoots | Butternut squash, | Avocado | Corn |
| Beet, 2 slices | ½ cup/60 grams | Beet, 4 slices | Okra |
| Bok choy, 3½ ounces | Cabbage, 3.5 ounces | Bok choy, 4½ ounces | Potato, sweet |
| Broccoli, ½ cup/1.6 | Cabbage, Savoy, | Broccoli, 1 cup/3.2 | Potato, white, all |
| ounces | ¾ cup | ounces | varieties |
| Brussels sprouts, | Leek, ½ /1½ ounces | Brussels sprouts, 6 | Seaweed |
| 2 sprouts | Parsnip | sprouts/4 ounces | Starch powder: |
| Cabbage: Savoy, | Peas, green, ⅓ cup | Cabbage, Savoy, 1 | arrowroot, corn, |
| ½ cup | Peppers, hot chili, | cup | potato, rice, tapioca |
| Carrot | less than 1½ | Cauliflower | Taro |
| Celery root/ Celeriac | ounces | Celery | Turnip |
| Chives | Spinach, 15 leaves | Fennel bulb, 1 cup; | Water chestnuts |
| Cucumber | Tomato, soup or juice | leaves, 3 cups | Yam |
| Eggplant | Tomato, Sun-dried, 2 | Garlic | Yucca |
| Endive | tablespoons | Jerusalem artichoke | |
| Fennel bulb, ½ cup, | | Leek, 1 leek/3 ounces | |
| leaves, 1 cup | | Mushrooms | |
| Green beans, 10 | | Onions | |
| beans/2½ ounces | | Peas, green, ½ cup | |
| Greens: lettuce, | | Scallions, white part | |
| collard, chard, kale, | | Shallot | |
| spinach | | Snow peas, 10 pods | |
| Olives | | Sugar snap peas | |
| Peas, green, ¼ cup | | Zucchini, ¾ cup | |
| Peppers, hot chili, 1 | | | |
| scant ounce | | | |
| Peppers, sweet bell | | | |
| Radicchio, 12 leaves | | | |
| Radish | | | |
| Rutabaga | | | |
| Scallion, green part | | | |
| only | | | |
| Snow peas, 5 pods | | | |
| Squash, butternut, | | | |
| ¼ cup, kabocha, | | | |
| sunburst, yellow | | | |

# FRUITS

LESS FERMENTABLE ————————————————→ MORE FERMENTABLE

| "Green Foods"— SCD Legal, LOW FODMAP | "Yellow Foods"— SCD Legal, MODERATE FODMAP | "Orange Foods"—SCD Legal, HIGH FODMAP | "Red Foods"—SCD Illegal, HIGH FODMAP |
|---|---|---|---|
| Tomato | Cherries, 3 | Apple | Jam/Jelly, commercial |
| Zucchini, ¾ cup | Cranberry, 1 | Apricot | Plantain |
| Banana, fresh or dried | tablespoon | Avocado | |
| Berries: blueberries, | Grapefruit, | Berries: cranberry, | |
| less than | ½ grapefruit | 2 tablespoons; | |
| 80 berries; | Honeydew melon, | blueberries, more | |
| boysenberry; | ½ cup/3½ ounces | than 80/100 grams; | |
| raspberry; | Longan, 10 | blackberries; | |
| strawberry, | Lychee, 5 | raspberries, more | |
| 10 pieces | Passion fruit, 4 pulps | than 50; cherries, 6 | |
| Carambola | Pineapple, dried, | Canned fruit in high | |
| Citrus: lemon, lime, | 1 slice | FODMAP fruit juice | |
| oranges, tangelos, | Rambutan, 4 | Currants, dried, | |
| tangerine | | 2 tablespoons | |
| Currant, dried, | | Custard Apple | |
| 1 tablespoon | | Date, dried | |
| Dragon Fruit | | Fig, dried | |
| Grapes | | Grapefruit, 1 | |
| Guava | | Mango* | |
| Jam/Jelly, homemade | | Nectarine | |
| (no pectin, sugar) | | Papaya, dried | |
| Kiwi | | Peach | |
| Longan, 5½ ounces | | Pear | |
| Melon: cantaloupe | | Pear, Asian | |
| (a.k.a. rockmelon), | | Persimmon | |
| honeydew, ½ cup/ | | Plum | |
| 3½ ounces | | Pomegranate, 1, | |
| Papaya/Paw Paw | | ½ cup seeds | |
| Passion fruit, 4 pulps | | Prunes | |
| Pineapple | | Raisins | |
| Pomegranate, | | Tamarillo* | |
| ½ pomegranate, | | Watermelon | |
| ¼ cup seeds | | | |
| Prickly Pear | | | |
| Rambutan, 2 | | | |
| Rhubarb | | | |

# LEGUMES AND BEANS

LESS FERMENTABLE → MORE FERMENTABLE

| "Green Foods"—SCD Legal, LOW FODMAP | "Yellow Foods"—SCD Legal, MODERATE FODMAP | "Orange Foods"—SCD Legal, HIGH FODMAP | "Red Foods"—SCD Illegal, HIGH FODMAP |
|---|---|---|---|
| Lentil, brown, ½ cup; green and red, ¼ cup | Black | Baked beans | Butter |
| Lima, ¼ cup | Lentil, green and red, ½ cup | Borlotti/Cranberry | Cannellini |
| | Lima, ⅓ cup | Kidney/Red | Chickpea/Garbanzo |
| | | Lima, ½ cup | Fava/Faba/Broad |
| | | Navy/White/Haricot | Pinto |
| | | Split peas | Soy |

# NUTS AND SEEDS

LESS FERMENTABLE → MORE FERMENTABLE

| "Green Foods"—SCD Legal, LOW FODMAP | "Yellow Foods"—SCD Legal, MODERATE FODMAP | "Orange Foods"—SCD Legal, HIGH FODMAP | "Red Foods"—SCD Illegal, HIGH FODMAP |
|---|---|---|---|
| Almonds, 10 nuts/ 0.42 ounces; flour, 2 tablespoons | Chestnuts, 1 handful | Almonds, 20 nuts; flour, ¼ cup | Chia seeds |
| Coconut: flour/ shredded, ¼ cup; milk (with no thickeners) | Flaxseed, less than 1 tablespoon | Cashews | Coconut milk with thickeners (guar gum, carrageenan) |
| Hazelnuts, 10 nuts | Hazelnuts, 20 nuts | Hazelnuts, 80 nuts | Seed flour |
| Macadamia, 20 nuts | Pecans, 40 nuts | Pine nuts, 8 tablespoons | |
| Peanut butter, 4 tablespoons | Walnuts, 3½ ounces | Pistachios | |
| Peanuts, 32 nuts | | Pumpkin seeds, 3½ ounces | |
| Pecans, 10 nuts | | Sesame seeds, 3½ ounces | |
| Pine nuts, 1 tablespoon | | Sunflower seeds, 3½ ounces | |
| Pumpkin seeds, 2 tablespoons | | | |
| Sesame seeds, 1 tablespoon | | | |
| Sunflower seeds, 2 teaspoons | | | |
| Walnuts, 10 nuts | | | |

# DAIRY

LESS FERMENTABLE ➜ MORE FERMENTABLE

| "Green Foods"— SCD Legal, LOW FODMAP | "Yellow Foods"— SCD Legal, MODERATE FODMAP | "Orange Foods"—SCD Legal, HIGH FODMAP | "Red Foods"—SCD Illegal, HIGH FODMAP |
|---|---|---|---|
| Butter<br>Cheese, aged more than 1 month; dry curd cottage cheese; yogurt cheese/labneh<br>Eggs<br>Ghee<br>Yogurt: homemade 24-hour | Cream: lactase-treated, ¼ cup<br>Milk: 100% Lactose-free | Yogurt: lactose-free commercial (pectin) | Cheese: cream cheese, cottage cheese, fresh cheese (feta, chevre, fresh mozzarella), ricotta<br>Cream<br>Kefir: commercial, homemade 24-hour<br>Milk<br>Sour cream: commercial<br>Yogurt: commercial |

# SWEETENERS

LESS FERMENTABLE ➜ MORE FERMENTABLE

| "Green Foods"— SCD Legal, LOW FODMAP | "Yellow Foods"— SCD Legal, MODERATE FODMAP | "Orange Foods"—SCD Legal, HIGH FODMAP | "Red Foods"—SCD Illegal, HIGH FODMAP |
|---|---|---|---|
| Aspartame, occasionally<br>Glucose/Dextrose<br>Honey: alfalfa, cotton, clover, raspberry, 2 tablespoons<br>Saccharine: pure (no high FODMAP or SCD illegal additives)<br>Stevia: pure (no inulin), in small amounts, occasionally | Honey*; blackberry, buckwheat, citrus/orange blossom, 1 tablespoon | Honey*; acacia, sage, tupelo | Agave syrup<br>Barley malt syrup<br>Brown rice syrup<br>Cane sugar (Rapadura, Sucanat)<br>Coconut sugar<br>Fructose, powdered<br>High-fructose corn syrup<br>Maple syrup<br>Molasses<br>Polyols/Sugar alcohol: isomalt, erythritol, lactitol, maltitol, mannitol, sorbitol, xylitol<br>Sucralose<br>Sugar/Sucrose |

# BEVERAGES AND ALCOHOL

LESS FERMENTABLE ➤ MORE FERMENTABLE

| "Green Foods"— SCD Legal, LOW FODMAP | "Yellow Foods"— SCD Legal, MODERATE FODMAP | "Orange Foods"—SCD Legal, HIGH FODMAP | "Red Foods"—SCD Illegal, HIGH FODMAP |
| --- | --- | --- | --- |
| **Common Drinks**<br>Coffee (weak), 1 cup per day<br>Cranberry juice, pure<br>Fruit juice from Low FODMAP fruits, ⅓ cup/3.4 ounces<br>Orange juice, fresh, ½ cup/4.2 ounces<br>Tea: black (weak), chamomile, ginger, green, hibiscus, lemongrass, mate, mint, oolong, rooibos/rooibos chai, rose hip<br>Water<br><br>**Alcohol**<br>Occasionally, in moderate amounts (See Note below):<br>Bourbon<br>Gin<br>Vodka<br>Whiskey/Scotch<br>Wine | **Common Drinks**<br>Seltzer/Carbonated beverages<br>Tea: green, less than 2 cups per day | **Common Drinks**<br>Fruit juice from high FODMAP fruits<br>Orange juice, 1 cup/ 4.2 ounces<br><br>**Alcohol**<br>Rum: light or gold* | **Common Drinks**<br>Coffee substitutes<br>Soda (fructose, sucrose)<br>Tea: chicory root, licorice, pau d'arco<br><br>**Alcohol**<br>Beer<br>Brandy<br>Hard cider<br>Liqueurs/Cordials<br>Rum: dark<br>Sherry<br>Tequila<br>Wine: dessert/sweet, sake, sparkling, port |

**Note:**
**Moderate amounts of alcohol are:**

Women—1 ounce per day, 3 to 5 times per week; Men—2½ ounces per day, 3 to 5 times per week

**Moderate amounts of wine are:**

Women—4 ounces per day, 3 to 5 times per week; Men—9 ounces per day, 3 to 5 times per week

## FATS AND OILS

LESS FERMENTABLE → MORE FERMENTABLE

| "Green Foods"—SCD Legal, LOW FODMAP | | | "Red Foods"—SCD Illegal, HIGH FODMAP |
|---|---|---|---|
| Butter | | | Soybean oil |
| Coconut oil | | | |
| Garlic-infused oil | | | |
| Ghee | | | |
| Macadamia oil | | | |
| Medium-chain triglyceride/MCT oil | | | |
| Olive oil | | | |
| Palm oil | | | |
| Polyunsaturated vegetable oils: Borage, Canola, Flax, Grape-seed, Hemp, Pumpkin seed, Sesame, Sunflower, Walnut | | | |

## SEASONINGS AND CONDIMENTS

LESS FERMENTABLE → MORE FERMENTABLE

| "Green Foods"—SCD Legal, LOW FODMAP | | | "Red Foods"—SCD Illegal, HIGH FODMAP |
|---|---|---|---|
| All spices except onion and garlic | | | Asafoetida powder |
| Garlic-infused oil | | | Chicory root, including leaves |
| Ginger, fresh and dried | | | Cocoa/chocolate, unsweetened |
| Mayonnaise, homemade or commercial with honey | | | Gums/Carrageenan/ Thickeners |
| Mustard, without garlic | | | Sauces or marinades with High FODMAP/ SCD Illegal items |
| Pickles/Relish, with no sweetener or garlic | | | Soy sauce/Tamari |
| Tabasco | | | Spices: Onion and garlic powder |
| Vinegar: apple cider, distilled white, red and white wine | | | Vinegar: balsamic |
| Wasabi, pure | | | |

# PROTEINS—TO ADD IF YOU WISH

LESS FERMENTABLE → MORE FERMENTABLE

| "Green Foods"—SCD Legal, LOW FODMAP | "Yellow Foods"—SCD Legal, MODERATE FODMAP | "Orange Foods"—SCD Legal, HIGH FODMAP | "Red Foods—SCD Illegal |
|---|---|---|---|
| Bacon, with honey<br>Beef<br>Broth: homemade meat or marrow bones (no cartilage)<br>Eggs<br>Fish<br>Game<br>Lamb<br>Organ meats<br>Pork<br>Poultry<br>Seafood | Bacon, w/sugar 1x per week | Broth: homemade bone/cartilage | Bacon, w/ high-fructose corn syrup<br>Deli/Processed meat with sugar, carrageenan, high FODMAP or SCD illegal additives<br>Note: While not included in the SSFG, firm tofu is low in FODMAPs and works for many people. |

# Acknowledgments

I never expected to be writing a book about digestive health, and I couldn't have done it without the knowledge and guidance of some very special experts. First and foremost, Dr. Allison Siebecker, who not only transformed my health but became a dear friend. Her contribution to SIBO healing has benefited thousands of people, and I hope this book further spreads her message. I have listened to hours of her teaching and am sharing what I have learned from her in this book. A special thank-you to her, also, for her medical review and consultations as I wrote this book. Dr. Mark Pimentel has also been incredibly generous with his time and knowledge, bringing light to a condition often overlooked by Western medical doctors. A special thank-you to SIBO nutritionist Kristy Regan for her insights and advice on the recipes in this book. Many other doctors and specialists have contributed their knowledge over the years—thank you to Dr. Mona Morstein, Dr. Nirala Jacobi, Dr. Gary Weiner, Dr. Steven Sandberg-Lewis, Dr. Rachel Fresco, Dr. Leonard Weinstock, Dr. Anne Hill, Dr. Michael Ruscio, Dr. Jason Hawrelak, Dr. Satish Rao, Dr. Lisa Shaver, Dr. Tom Messinger, Dr. Tom O'Bryan, Dr. Ami Kapadia, Dr. Ken Brown, Dr. Megan Taylor, Dr. Melanie Keller, Dr. Ilana Gurevich, Dr. Ali Rezaie, Dr. Sam Rahbar, Dr. Christine Schaffner, Dr. Suzanne Breen, Dr. Greg Nigh, Dr. Norm Robillard, Dr. Eric Zielinski, Dr. William Salt,

Dr. Ritamarie Loscalzo, Dr. Robyn Kutka, Dr. Sheila Dean, Gary Stapleton, Eric Hamilton, Rebecca Coomes, Kiran Krishnan, Larry Wurn, Ocean Robbins, Donna Gates, Jen Fugo, Kayle Sandberg-Lewis, Summer Bock, Christine Faler, Steve Wright, Jordan Reasoner, Angela Pifer, Maria Zilka, Mindy Tobin, Lisa Letizio, Sabrina Zielinski, Mary Agnes Antonopoulos, and Vonabell Sherman. Thank you to Karen Cook and Miles Larsen, who have been with me since Shivan's Yoga Studio and have given their time and love to this project. Thank you to my team: Cyndi Athmanathan, Lisa Nelson, and Mariel Urner. Thank you to Judy Kern, who was so helpful in making this book come to life.

I also want to thank the entire SIBO SOS community, who have inspired and encouraged me to make helping those with SIBO one of my life's work! What started as a passion project has become multiple online courses (including the SIBO Recovery Roadmap course with Dr. Allison Siebecker), expert Masterclasses, the *Digestion SOS: Rescue and Relief for IBS, SIBO, and Leaky Gut* docuseries, four SIBO Summits, and much more.

And, of course, thank you to my husband, David, for unwavering support through this process. Finally, thank you to Linda Bennett, my second mom and spiritual teacher, who has always believed in me, encouraged me, and pushed me to be my best. I couldn't and wouldn't have done this work without you.

# Index

Note: Page numbers in *italics* refer to graphs and charts.